BMA

Fast Facts:
Chemotherapy-
Induced Nausea
& Vomiting

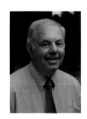

Rudolph M Navari MD

Director, Cancer Care Program

Central and South America

World Health Organization

Professor, Indiana University School of Medicine South Bend

South Bend, Indiana, USA

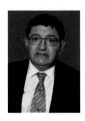

Bernardo L Rapoport MD

Specialist Physician and Medical Oncologist-in-Charge

The Medical Oncology Centre of Rosebank

Saxonwold

Johannesburg

South Africa

D1420158

Declaration of Independenc

This book is as balanced and a:

Ideas for improvement are alwa

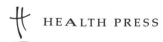

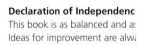

1000572

HEALTH PRESS

Fast Facts: Chemotherapy-Induced Nausea and Vomiting
First published April 2016

Text © 2016 Rudolph M Navari, Bernardo L Rapoport
© 2016 in this edition Health Press Limited

Health Press Limited, Elizabeth House, Queen Street, Abingdon,
Oxford OX14 3LN, UK.
Tel: +44 (0)1235 523233

Book orders can be placed by telephone or via the website.

For regional distributors or to order via the website, please go to:
fastfacts.com

For telephone orders, please call +44 (0)1752 202301 (UK, Europe and Asia–
Pacific), 1 800 247 6553 (USA, toll free) or +1 419 281 1802 (Americas).

Fast Facts is a trademark of Health Press Limited.

The publisher and the authors have made every effort to ensure the accuracy of this
book, but cannot accept responsibility for any errors or omissions.

For all drugs, please consult the product labeling approved in your country for
prescribing information.

Registered names, trademarks, etc. used in this book, even when not marked as
such, are not to be considered unprotected by law.

A CIP record for this title is available from the British Library.

ISBN 978-1-910797-11-2

Navari R (Rudolph) M
Fast Facts: Chemotherapy-Induced Nausea and Vomiting/
Rudolph M Navari, Bernardo L Rapoport

Medical illustrations by Annamaria Dutto, Withernsea, UK.
Typesetting by User Design, Illustration and Typesetting, Leicester, UK.
Printed in Europe with Xpedient Print.

List of abbreviations

5-HT$_3$ receptor: 5-hydroxytryptamine-3 (serotonin) receptor

AC chemotherapy: anthracycline and cyclophosphamide chemotherapy

CINV: chemotherapy-induced nausea and vomiting

CTZ: chemotherapy trigger zone

GABA: γ-aminobutyric acid

GI: gastrointestinal

HEC: highly emetogenic chemotherapy

MEC: moderately emetogenic chemotherapy

NK-1: neurokinin-1

NTS: nucleus tractus solitarius

RA: receptor antagonist

VC: vomiting center

Introduction

Few side effects of cancer treatment are more feared by the patient than nausea and vomiting. Although chemotherapy-induced nausea and vomiting (CINV) is not life threatening, it is associated with a significant deterioration in quality of life. CINV can result in severely debilitating weakness, weight loss, electrolyte imbalance, dehydration or anorexia, and is associated with a variety of complications, including fractures, esophageal tears, decline in behavioral and mental status, and wound dehiscence. Furthermore, it can often result in patients refusing further courses of chemotherapy.

Failure to control acute CINV on the first day of chemotherapy increases the risk of CINV on subsequent days and in subsequent cycles of chemotherapy. Health professionals tend to underestimate the number of patients with delayed CINV as, once discharged, patients often do not report the side effects of treatment that they experience at home. When they do, additional supportive care such as intravenous hydration and antiemetics, and the increased risk of hospitalization can have a large enconomic impact on healthcare systems.

Over the past two decades, very effective agents have been developed for the prevention of CINV along with clear international guidelines on their use. However, clinicians are too often unaware of the proper prophylaxis required to protect their patients from CINV in both inpatient and outpatient settings.

Fast Facts: Chemotherapy-Induced Nausea and Vomiting presents the evidence for the clinical agents available for the prevention of CINV, and recommendations for their use in various clinical settings using recently established guidelines.

Prevention of CINV ensures a better quality of life for patients both during and after treatment, and improves adherence to subsequent cancer treatments, often resulting in better long-term outcomes. For all health professionals in a position to make this kind of a difference, this is the book for you!

Definitions

It is estimated that 80–100% of patients receiving chemotherapy without antiemetic prophylaxis will experience some level of chemotherapy-induced nausea and vomiting (CINV). The sensation of nausea and the act of vomiting are protective reflexes that rid the intestine and stomach of toxic substances.

Nausea. The experience of nausea is subjective. It is a difficult-to-describe sick or queasy sensation, usually perceived as being in the stomach. Nausea and vomiting are not necessarily on a continuum. Although nausea may be considered a prodromal phase to the act of vomiting, patients may experience significant nausea without vomiting.[1] Conversely, patients may have sudden emesis without nausea. Nausea has been assumed to be the conscious awareness of unusual sensations in the 'vomiting center' of the brainstem (see below), but the existence of such a center and its relationship to nausea remain controversial.[1]

Vomiting consists of a pre-ejection phase called retching, and ejection, and is accompanied by shivering and salivation.

Pathophysiology

The mechanisms of nausea and vomiting are not well defined. Vomiting is a reflex activated by toxic substances such as chemotherapy drugs, which may directly affect areas in the cerebral cortex and the medulla oblongata, or may stimulate the small intestine via the vagus nerve. Afferent impulses, triggered from the cerebral cortex, chemoreceptor trigger zone (CTZ), pharynx and vagal afferent fibers of the gastrointestinal (GI) tract, then travel to the vomiting center (VC) – termed the 'central pattern generator' by some authors[2] – in the lateral reticular formation of the medulla (Figure 1.1).

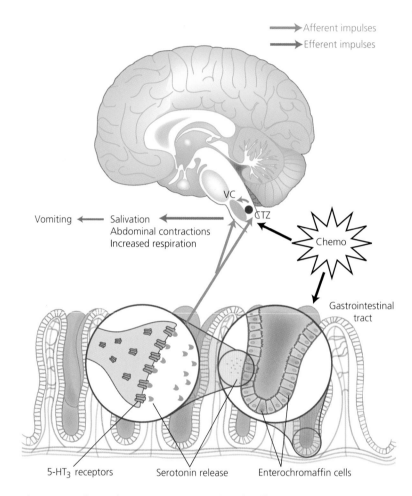

Figure 1.1 Chemotherapy agents may directly affect the chemoreceptor trigger zone (CTZ) in the medulla oblongata or may stimulate the small intestine via the vagus nerve. Damage caused by chemotherapy to enterochromaffin cells in the gastrointestinal (GI) tract releases serotonin. The serotonin binds to vagal afferent receptors in the bowel wall, sending afferent impulses from the GI tract to the vomiting center (VC) in the brain, which is sensitive to several neurotransmitters (serotonin, dopamine, substance P). Activation of the VC, either directly or indirectly through the CTZ, produces efferent impulses that increase salivation and respiratory rate and cause pharngeal, GI and abdominal muscle contractions, resulting in vomiting.[4]

The VC is the primary structure that coordinates the mechanisms of nausea and vomiting; it is sensitive to several neurotransmitters (serotonin, dopamine, substance P), which are released through these pathways.[1] Each individual may require a different level of stimulation to the VC to reach the threshold for nausea or vomiting, such that individuals will experience different responses to the same stimuli.[5]

The mechanism that is best supported by research involves an effect on the upper small intestine. When rapidly dividing enterochromaffin cells in the GI tract are damaged, serotonin is released and binds to vagal afferent receptors in the wall of the bowel that activate the VC and stimulate emesis either directly or indirectly through the CTZ. The CTZ is situated in the area postrema of the medulla near the fourth ventricle.[2] It is strongly suspected that the nucleus tractus solitarius (NTS) neurons, which lie ventrally to the area postrema, initiate emesis.[6] This medullary area is a convergence point for projections arising from the area postrema and the vestibular and vagal afferent. The NTS is a good candidate for the site of action of centrally acting antiemetics.

Activation of the VC produces efferent impulses that travel from the VC to the abdominal muscles, salivation center, cranial nerves and respiratory center, causing vomiting. Nausea is thought to be mediated by the autonomic nervous system.

Control of CINV. The main approach to the control of emesis has been to identify the active neurotransmitters (Figure 1.2) and their receptors in the CNS and the GI tract that mediate the afferent inputs to the VC. The receptors associated with serotonin and substance P are 5-hydroxytryptamine-3 (5-HT_3) and neurokinin-1 (NK-1), respectively. The study of these serotonin and substance P receptors has guided the development of antagonists, with relative success in controlling emesis (Table 1.1) (also see Chapter 3).

Despite some reduction of nausea after treatment with 5HT_3 and NK-1 receptor antagonists (RAs), it remains a problem, suggesting other pathways may be important in controlling nausea.

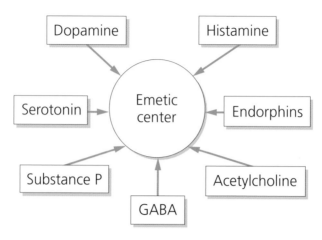

Figure 1.2 Neurotransmitters involved in the mechanism of emesis. GABA, γ-aminobutyric acid.

TABLE 1.1

Antiemetic receptor antagonists

Dopamine RAs	5-HT$_3$ RAs	Dopa-5-HT$_3$ RAs	NK-1 RAs
Butyrophenones	Azasetron	Metoclopramide	Aprepitant (MK-869)
Olanzapine	Dolasetron*		
Phenothiazines	Granisetron[†]		Fosaprepitant
	Ondansetron		Netupitant
	Palonosetron		Rolapitant
	Ramosetron		
	Tropisetron		

*Not recommended in the USA (FDA). [†]Intravenous dose restriction in the USA (FDA). 5-HT$_3$, serotonin; NK-1 neurokinin-1; RA, receptor antagonist.

Dopamine RAs have been shown to have some efficacy in the treatment of nausea and vomiting caused by chemotherapy. They have not been effective in the prevention of CINV. Agents that may affect γ-aminobutyric acid (GABA), histaminic and muscarinic receptors are also being investigated with a view to developing additional effective antiemetic drugs.

Dopaminergic, histaminic and muscarinic receptors may be some of the receptors involved in the control of nausea.[7,8]

Key points – definitions and pathophysiology

- It is estimated that 80–100% of patients receiving chemotherapy without antiemetic prophylaxis will experience some level of chemotherapy-induced nausea and vomiting.
- Nausea and vomiting are triggered when afferent impulses from the cerebral cortex, chemoreceptor trigger zone (CTZ), pharynx and vagal afferent fibers of the gastrointestinal (GI) tract travel to the vomiting center (VC) in the central nervous system.
- The main approach to the control of emesis has been to identify the active neurotransmitters (serotonin and substance P) and their receptors (5-hydroxytryptamine-3 [5-HT$_3$] and neurokinin-1 [NK-1]) in the CNS and the GI tract that mediate the afferent inputs to the VC.
- Several 5-HT$_3$ and NK-1 receptor antagonists have been developed for the prevention of chemotherapy-induced emesis.

Key references

1. Stern RM, Koch KL, Andrews PLR, eds. *Nausea: Mechanisms and Management.* New York: Oxford University Press, 2011.

2. Koga T, Fukuda H. Neurons in the nucleus of the solitary tract mediating inputs from vagal afferents and the area postrema in the pattern generator in the emetic act in dogs. *Neurosci Res* 1992;14:366–79.

3. Hesketh PJ. Chemotherapy-induced nausea and vomiting. *N Engl J Med* 2008;358:2482–94.

4. Hesketh PJ, Van Belle S, Aapro M et al. Differential involvement of neurotransmitters through the time course of cisplatin-induced emesis as revealed by therapy with specific receptor antagonists. *Eur J Cancer* 2003;39:1074–80.

5. Hockenberry-Eaton M, Benner A. Patterns of nausea and vomiting in children: Nursing assessment and intervention. *Oncol Nurs Forum* 1990;17:575–84.

6. Yates BJ, Grelot L, Kerman IA et al. Organization of the vestibular inputs to nucleus tractus solitarius and adjacent structures in cat brain stem. *Am J Physiol* 1994;267: R974–83.

7. Navari RM. Management of chemotherapy-induced nausea and vomiting: focus on new agents and new uses for older agents. *Drugs* 2013;73:249–62.

8. Navari RM. Treatment of chemotherapy-induced nausea. *Community Oncol* 2012;9:20–6.

Types of chemotherapy-induced nausea and vomiting

Five categories are used to classify CINV (Figure 2.1):
- acute
- delayed
- breakthrough
- refractory
- anticipatory.

Nausea and vomiting may occur any time after the administration of chemotherapy, but the mechanisms appear different for CINV that occurs in the first 24 hours after chemotherapy compared with CINV that occurs 1–5 days after chemotherapy (Table 2.1).[1]

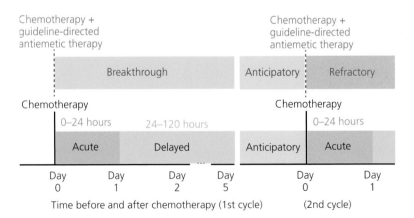

Figure 2.1 Timing of the different types of chemotherapy-induced nausea and vomiting (CINV). Acute and delayed nausea and vomiting occur after chemotherapy when no antiemetic treatment is given. Breakthrough and refractory CINV occur despite guideline-directed antiemetic therapy. Anticipatory CINV is attributed to the adverse memory of previous CINV whether or not antiemetics have been given.

TABLE 2.1

The timing and mechanisms of the different types of chemotherapy-induced nausea and vomiting

Category	Time interval	Mechanism
Acute	First 24 hours after chemotherapy	Serotonin receptors in GI tract
Delayed	24–120 hours after chemotherapy	Neurokinin-1 receptors in CNS
Breakthrough	0–120 hours after chemotherapy	Unknown
Refractory	CINV in subsequent chemotherapy cycles	Unknown
Anticipatory	Nausea and vomiting in anticipation of scheduled chemotherapy	Psychological; anxiety

CNS, central nervous system; GI, gastrointestinal.

Acute CINV is nausea and/or vomiting that occurs within the first 24 hours of chemotherapy administration. It can start within 1 or 2 hours of chemotherapy being administered and can last for several hours, with maximal intensity 5–6 hours after drug administration. The incidence (see page 19)[2], severity and quantity of acute emesis and/or nausea varies depending on several treatment-related factors including the emetogenicity and dosage of the chemotherapy (see Chapter 4) and a number of patient-related factors (see Risk factors below).[1]

Delayed CINV is arbitrarily defined as nausea and/or vomiting that develops more than 24 hours after chemotherapy administration. It is important to emphasize that there is no clear break for when acute CINV ends and delayed CINV starts and the definitions for both should be considered an approximation.

Delayed CINV is typically associated with the administration of cisplatin, doxorubicin or cyclophosphamide and can occur days 2 to 7 after chemotherapy. It can persist for as long as 5–7 days, with maximal intensity 48–72 hours after drug administration. It is more common in those who experience acute emesis/nausea.

Other predictive factors include the dose and the emetogenicity of the chemotherapeutic agent (see Chapter 4), patient sex and age, and protection against nausea and vomiting in previous cycles of chemotherapy.[1] For cisplatin, which has been most extensively studied, delayed emesis reaches peak intensity 2–3 days after chemotherapy administration and can last up to a week if not treated.[1, 3–6]

Breakthrough CINV is vomiting and/or nausea that occurs within 5 days of chemotherapy despite appropriate guideline-directed use of prophylactic antiemetic agents. This type of CINV usually requires immediate treatment or 'rescue' treatment with additional antiemetics.

Refractory CINV is vomiting and/or nausea that occurs after chemotherapy in subsequent chemotherapy cycles when guideline-directed antiemetic prophylaxis and/or rescue treatment have failed in earlier cycles.[1]

Anticipatory CINV. Patients who experience CINV may develop a conditioned response known as anticipatory nausea and/or vomiting before the administration of chemotherapy in future chemotherapy cycles. This is attributed to the adverse memory of previous CINV. Incidence rates for this type of nausea and vomiting range from 10% to 45%, with nausea occurring more frequently.[1, 3–6] Anticipatory CINV can be triggered by a variety of tastes, odors, sights, thoughts or anxiety associated with the chemotherapy treatment. It is more challenging to control and treat than acute or delayed CINV.

Risk factors

Risk factors for CINV include features of the treatment itself as well as a number of patient characteristics.

Treatment risk factors. The potential for CINV may be influenced by the following features of the chemotherapy being administered:
- the emetogenicity of chemotherapy agents (see Tables 4.1 and 4.2, pages 54–7)
- the doses of chemotherapy administered (see Table 4.3, page 59)
- the route of administration (see Table 4.1, page 54)
- the infusion duration
- the combination of chemotherapy agents.

Patient characteristics also influence the potential for CINV (Table 2.2).[1] Young women with a history of motion sickness, emesis during pregnancy and no history of alcohol consumption

TABLE 2.2

Patient-related risk factors for emesis following chemotherapy

Major factors	Minor factors
• Female sex	• History of motion sickness
• Age < 50 years	• History of emesis during past pregnancy
• History of prior low chronic alcohol intake (< 1 ounce of alcohol/day)	• Anxiety
• History of previous chemotherapy-induced emesis	

have the highest risk of developing significant CINV. These patients should receive the most effective prophylactic antiemetic regimen available based on the international antiemetic guidelines (see Chapter 4).

Incidence in high-risk patients. Despite the use of guideline-directed prophylactic antiemetics, CINV can occur with relatively high frequency in high-risk patients (20–25% acute, 50–70% delayed, 50% breakthrough and 30% refractory).

Patients who are scheduled to receive their first course of chemotherapy should be individually evaluated for their specific risk factors and prescribed appropriate antiemetics (see Chapter 7).

Treatment effectiveness

The use of antiemetic agents, as recommended by international guidelines, has been shown to prevent emesis in approximately 50–70% of patients receiving either highly or moderately emetogenic chemotherapy.[3-6] The prevention of nausea has been much less successful with currently approved agents.[7,8] New agents and new combinations of agents are necessary to adequately prevent chemotherapy-induced nausea.

Differential diagnosis

Although the onset and duration of symptoms usually points to chemotherapy as the cause, other potential aggravating factors that may cause nausea and vomiting in patients with cancer should be considered (Table 2.3). Immunocompromised and elderly patients are more vulnerable to infections and should be evaluated for bacterial or viral gastroenteritis.

TABLE 2.3

Differential diagnoses

Structural

- Bowel obstruction
- Hepatosplenomegaly
- Brain metastasis
- Increased intracranial pressure
- Inner ear problems
- Urinary tract infection

Psychological

- Anxiety
- Depression
- Uncontrolled pain

Treatment

- Opioids
- Antidepressants
- Antibiotics (e.g. erythromycin)
- Abdominopelvic radiotherapy

Metabolic

- Hypo/hypernatremia
- Hypo/hyperkalemia
- Hypercalcemia

Key points – types of CINV and risk factors

- The different types of CINV are classified according to the time interval at which nausea and vomiting occurs in relation to the administration of chemotherapy.
- Chemotherapy agents vary in their emetogenicity; for example, cisplatin has high emetogenic potential and causes CINV in almost all patients who do not receive antiemetic prophylaxis.
- Important individual patient characteristics contribute to the risk of developing CINV.
- Despite guideline-directed antiemetic prophylaxis, CINV can occur with relatively high frequency in high-risk patients (20–25% acute CINV, 50–70% delayed CINV, 50% breakthrough CINV and 30% refractory CINV).
- The guideline-directed use of antiemetic agents has been shown to prevent emesis in approximately 50–70% of patients receiving highly or moderately emetogenic chemotherapy.
- The prevention of nausea has been much less successful with currently approved agents.

Key references

1. Navari RM. Management of chemotherapy-induced nausea and vomiting: focus on new agents and new uses for older agents. *Drugs* 2013;73:249–62.

2. Cohen L, de Moor CA, Eisenberg P et al. Chemotherapy-induced nausea and vomiting: incidence and impact on patient quality of life at community oncology settings. *Support Care Cancer* 2007;15:497–503.

3. Roila F, Herrstedt J, Aapro M et al. Guideline update for MASCC and ESMO in the prevention of chemotherapy- and radiotherapy-induced nausea and vomiting: results of the Perugia consensus conference. *Ann Oncol* 2010;21:232–43.

4. Basch E, Prestrud AA, Hesketh PJ et al. Antiemetic American Society Clinical Oncology clinical practice guideline update. *J Clin Oncol* 2011;29:4189–98.

5. Hesketh PJ, Bohike K, Lyman GH et al. Antiemetics: American Society of Clinical Oncology focused guideline update. *J Clin Oncol* 2016;34:381–6.

6. NCCN Clinical Practice Guidelines in Oncology version 1 2015. Antiemesis. National Comprehensive Cancer Network (NCCN) [online]. www.nccn.org/professionals/physician_gls/PDF/antiemesis.pdf, last accessed October 2015.

7. Ng TL, Hutton B, Clemons M. Chemotherapy-induced nausea and vomiting: time for more emphasis on nausea? *Oncologist* 2015;20:576–83.

8. Navari RM. Treatment of chemotherapy-induced nausea. *Community Oncol* 2012;9:20–6.

Significant advances have been made in the development of agents to control chemotherapy-induced nausea and vomiting (CINV) over the past two decades thanks to a better understanding of the physiological and molecular pathways underlying CINV (see Chapter 1) and knowledge of the different responses individuals have to chemotherapy (see Chapter 2). As a result, major progress has been made in the treatment of patients with cancer undergoing chemotherapy. Recent developments in antiemetic research have expanded the roles of the various classes of drugs and the optimal combinations of available agents, resulting in more available treatment options for CINV.

A historical perspective

In the early 1990s, treatment for CINV included the corticosteroid dexamethasone. Management was further improved by the use of agents that disrupt signals from the brain, sent by specific neurotransmitters that cause nausea and vomiting, to matching receptors in the body. In particular, the discovery of the 5-hydroxytryptamine (5-HT$_3$) receptor and the development of 5-HT$_3$ receptor antagonists (RAs) (ondansetron, granisetron, tropisetron, dolasetron, palonosetron) significantly advanced the treatment of CINV. CINV control was further improved by combining the 5-HT$_3$ RAs with dexamethasone.

Over the past decade, discovery of the role of the neurokinin-1 (NK-1) receptor in the pathogenesis of delayed CINV and the development of NK-1 RAs (aprepitant, netupitant, rolapitant) have led to significant developments in the management of emetogenic anticancer treatment.

Despite these milestone achievements, nausea in particular (60% of patients), and vomiting (30% of patients) remain clinically significant problems for patients undergoing highly emetogenic chemotherapy (HEC) and moderately emetogenic chemotherapy (MEC). The effect of CINV on patients' quality of life can be devastating, and patients who experience uncontrollable nausea and vomiting associated with their therapy may be reluctant to continue with additional chemotherapy. Proper administration of antiemetics reduces CINV and improves patients' quality of life, such that patients are more likely to undergo subsequent chemotherapy cycles.

Administering the correct receptor antagonist

Serotonin, substance P and dopamine are the key neurotransmitters sent from the chemoreceptor trigger zone (CTZ) and gastrointestinal tract that elicit the CINV response (see page 11; Figure 1.1). These neurotransmitters and their receptors operate via different signaling mechanisms (see below), which is why it is important to administer the correct receptor antagonist.

Signaling mechanisms. Serotonin ($5\text{-}HT_3$) is the main mediator of neural signals from the gut to the CNS. $5\text{-}HT_3$ RAs compete with serotonin for binding to serotonin-type 3 receptors in the gut wall, thereby blocking a proemetic signal to the CNS and suppressing the patient's urge to vomit. The newest $5\text{-}HT_3$ RA, palonosetron, has a higher receptor-binding ability than other commonly used $5\text{-}HT_3$ RAs, which may make it more effective at preventing CINV.

Substance P transmits signals from the vagus nerve to NK-1 receptors in the CTZ and the gut. NK-1 RAs compete with substance P for binding to these NK-1 receptors. Clinically, administration of aprepitant, the first drug to antagonize the NK-1 receptor, has proven effective in preventing delayed CINV when combined with $5\text{-}HT_3$ RA and corticosteroids.

The role of dopamine is less clear, but dopamine release and cognate dopamine receptor-2 signaling is known to play an important role in the pathogenesis of CINV, and dopamine antagonists have been shown to be effective in treating CINV.

Time of action. Substance P and serotonin are thought to have different time courses of action that correspond to the biphasic nature of emesis caused by cisplatin-based HEC (Figure 3.1).

The 5-HT$_3$-mediated effect happens within a few hours of the administration of chemotherapy, early in the acute phase. It has a short duration of action; virtually complete in the first 24 hours after chemotherapy adminstration. The substance P-mediated effect starts roughly 15 hours after chemotherapy administration and extends into the delayed phase. It continues for 60–96 hours after the administration of HEC.

The acute phase of chemotherapy has been arbitrarily determined as the initial 24 hours after chemotherapy infusion, and the delayed phase defined as any time in the 96 hours after the acute phase (24–120 hours after chemotherapy). It is important to point out that these 'acute' 'delayed' phase definitions are based on the need for readily measurable endpoints, rather than the biological aspects associated with serotonin and NK-1 or substance P. However, the NK-1 RA and 5-HT$_3$ RA are associated with acute and delayed CINV, respectively.

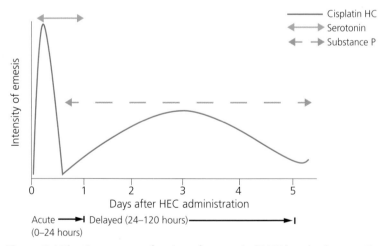

Figure 3.1 The time course of action of serotonin (5-HT$_3$) and substance P correspond to the biphasic pattern of emesis associated with highly emetogenic chemotherapy (HEC), i.e. the acute and delayed phases of CINV.[1,2]

5-Hydroxytryptamine-3 receptor antagonists

Granisetron (endo-N-[9 -methyl-9-aza- bicyclo-(3.3.1) non-3-ylI1-methyl-1H-indazole-3-car- boxamide hydrochloride) is a highly selective 5-HT$_3$ RA, available as an intravenous, oral and transdermal preparation for the treatment of CINV.

Dosage. Intravenous granisetron, 10 µg/kg, is administered over 5 minutes within 30 minutes of the start of chemotherapy treatment. International guidelines recommend that 5-HT$_3$ RAs be given only on the day of chemotherapy. The oral dose is 1–2 mg/day.

Efficacy in acute CINV. Development of granisetron began in 1985 and clinical trials were initiated in 1987. In all the clinical trials of granisetron for CINV, a complete responder was defined as a patient who experienced 'no vomiting and no, or only mild, nausea' in the first 24 hours after chemotherapy. This differs from the complete response criteria used in the clinical trials of other 5-HT$_3$ RAs – ondansetron and tropisetron studies used 'no vomiting' as the only complete response criterion making comparisons between clinical trials in this class of drug complex. The use of 'no vomiting' as the only criterion for 'complete' control can be misleading, because a particular patient could feel very nauseous yet still be assessed as a complete responder.

Granisetron has demonstrated significant activity in patients receiving both cisplatin and non-cisplatin treatment.[3,4] The first double-blind placebo-controlled study was conducted in 28 patients with cancer receiving cisplatin chemotherapy (mean dose > 80 mg/m^2); they were given either a single intravenous dose of granisetron, 40 µg/kg, or placebo. Granisetron demonstrated significant efficacy; following a 5-minute infusion, 93% of patients remained free from significant nausea and vomiting (complete response), compared with 7% in the placebo group. In addition, 93% of patients in the placebo group required rescue therapy with granisetron, 40 µg/kg. After a single rescue dose, all patients showed resolution or improvement of symptoms within a few minutes of infusion.[5]

Two large single-blind (patient-blind) multicenter studies compared the activity of granisetron with that of metoclopramide, 7 mg/kg, plus dexamethasone, 12 mg, in patients receiving high-dose cisplatin chemotherapy, and with that of chlorpromazine, 25 mg, plus dexamethasone, 12 mg, in patients receiving non-cisplatin chemotherapy. A complete response to prophylaxis with granisetron, 40 µg/kg, in the control of acute emesis was observed in 70% of patients in each trial.[6,7] Furthermore, granisetron was statistically better than the metoclopramide–dexamethasone combination.

Several double-blind dose-finding studies with a total of 1735 patients receiving cisplatin and non-cisplatin therapy also demonstrated that a single dose of granisetron, 40 µg/kg, or 3 mg in a 75-kg person, provided optimal control of CINV.

Efficacy over repeated chemotherapy cycles. An optimal antiemetic must maintain control of nausea and vomiting over multiple cycles of chemotherapy. Before the development of the 5-HT$_3$ RAs, several studies had noted that the efficacy of antiemetics decreased over successive cycles of treatment. A study that examined whether the efficacy of intravenous granisetron was maintained over successive cycles found that, with either 3 mg or 40 µg/kg dosing, approximately 60% of patients were complete responders for up to 8 cycles.[8]

Efficacy over multiple-day chemotherapy cycles. Some chemotherapeutic regimens are highly emetogenic. One way to decrease the emetic burden is to divide or fractionate the therapy over multiple days. This strategy is used for the treatment of particular types of cancer such as testicular cancer and teratoma. The effectiveness of granisetron in the management of nausea and vomiting induced by multiple-day chemotherapy was evaluated in two comparative studies comprising 481 patients. Patients received their first course of chemotherapy (cisplatin, ifosfamide or etoposide) divided over 5 days. Intravenous granisetron, 40 µg/kg, was compared with metoclopramide plus dexamethasone in one study and with alizapride plus dexamethasone in the other. Granisetron was superior on day 1 in both trials. In addition, the proportion of complete responders over the 5-day period was greater for granisetron than for the comparators (54% vs 42.7% alizapride plus dexamethasone; 46.8% vs 43.9% metoclopramide plus dexamethasone).[9]

Efficacy in delayed CINV. Conventional antiemetics do not control delayed nausea and vomiting adequately. Combinations such as dexamethasone plus metoclopramide, for example, have shown only marginal benefits. The efficacy of a single dose of intravenous granisetron, 40 µg/kg or 3 mg, was assessed in a multicenter study over a 7-day period, with 533 patients receiving cisplatin chemotherapy (275 mg/m^2).

Granisetron was shown to be beneficial in both the acute (day 1) and to some degree the late (days 5–7) phases of cisplatin-induced nausea and vomiting, but was not effective between days 2 and 4. Cisplatin-induced nausea and vomiting is a biphasic event, with emesis possibly mediated by non-5-HT$_3$ receptor-based mechanisms during the early delayed phase (days 2–4) and late delayed phase (days 5–7). Minor relief from delayed nausea and vomiting was observed with granisetron.

Approximately half of patients receiving granisetron who were treated with doses of less than 75 mg/m^2 cisplatin experienced delayed CINV, compared with two-thirds of those treated with 75–100 mg/m^2 and 80% of those receiving more than 100 mg/m^2. Similarly, in a trial using an antiemetic regimen of dexamethasone plus metoclopramide, fewer patients receiving less than 90 mg/m^2 of cisplatin were diagnosed with delayed nausea and vomiting than those receiving high-dose cisplatin (90 mg/m^2).

Safety and tolerability. Granisetron has an excellent safety profile. Granisetron administered at doses as high as seven times the standard clinical dose (up to 300 µg/kg) causes no significant toxicity. Headache and constipation are the most common side effects. Headaches are treatable with simple analgesics, and constipation often resolves spontaneously. In unusual cases, constipation has required treatment with enemas or laxatives.

Transdermal granisetron. Granisetron transdermal delivery system (granisetron TDS) is a slow-release patch containing 34.3 mg of granisetron, delivering 3.1 mg per 24 hours. It is indicated for the prevention of CINV in patients receiving MEC or HEC regimens of up to 5 consecutive days. It is a convenient alternative route for delivering granisetron for up to 7 days

Transdermal drug delivery systems provide systemic treatment by passive diffusion through the skin. This alternative route of administration may be well suited for patients who are unable to take oral treatments, and has the potential of improving patient adherence to treatment.

Efficacy and tolerability. In a double-blind phase III trial that compared both efficacy and tolerability, 641 patients were randomized to oral granisetron, 2 mg/day for 3–5 days, or granisetron TDS, one patch for 7 days, before receiving multi-day chemotherapy. The primary endpoint of the study was complete control of CINV (no vomiting/retching, no more than mild nausea, no rescue medication) from the start of chemotherapy until 24 hours after final administration. Granisetron TDS demonstrated non-inferiority (prespecified margin of 15%) to oral granisetron, with complete control attained in 60% of patients (versus 65% in the oral group). Both treatments were well tolerated, with constipation the most common side effect.[10]

The most common adverse reaction with granisetron TDS is constipation (5.4%). The incidence of headaches is low (0.7%). Application site reactions in the form of pain, pruritus, erythema, rash, irritation, vesicles, burn, discoloration and urticaria may occur in a few patients. Patch non-adhesion is very uncommon.

APF350 is an injectable extended-release long-acting formulation of granisetron for the prevention of CINV. APF350 has been shown to maintain therapeutic drug levels of granisetron for at least 5 days after a single subcutaneous injection. This product is currently in research and is not yet licensed. It may be commercially available in the future.

Efficacy and tolerability of APF350 has been studied as part of a three-drug regimen with the intravenous NK-1 RA fosaprepitant and the intravenous/oral corticosteroid dexamethasone. The primary endpoint was attained in the multicenter placebo-controlled phase III MAGIC trial (Modified Absorption Granisetron In the Prevention of CINV), in patients receiving HEC regimens. The percentage of patients who achieved a complete response in the delayed phase was significantly higher in the APF350 arm than the comparator arm (64.7% vs 56.6%). Adverse events were generally mild to moderate in severity and of short duration.[11]

In a phase III study involving more than 1300 patients, APF350 demonstrated statistical non-inferiority to palonosetron in the prevention of acute and delayed CINV with MEC and acute CINV with HEC.[12]

Injection site reactions are the most commonly reported adverse events for APF350.

Ondansetron ([+]1,2,3,9-tetrahydro-9-methyl-3-[2-methyl-1H-imidazol-1-yl] methyl-4H-carbazol-4-one monohydrochloride dihydrate) was originally researched for the management of patients with migraine. The product was subsequently investigated and approved as an intravenous and oral antiemetic for CINV.

Dosage. The recommended intravenous dosage is 16 mg infused over 15 minutes. Treatment should begin 30 minutes before the start of chemotherapy, and the first treatment is usually infused over 15 minutes. The oral dosage is 8-mg three times daily, with the first tablet given 30 minutes before the start of chemotherapy, followed by 8 mg every 8 hours for 1–2 days after completion of chemotherapy.

Efficacy in acute CINV. The original clinical data on ondansetron in CINV appeared in 1987 in a study of

15 patients receiving non-cisplatin cytotoxic drugs of moderate or mild emetogenic potential, including an anthracycline, cyclophosphamide, vincristine, epirubicin, mitoxantrone, methotrexate, doxorubicin, etoposide and 5-fluorouracil, given in various combinations. Ondansetron, 16 mg, given as an initial intravenous dose of 4 mg followed by three 4-mg oral doses, provided total protection from CINV in 14 of the 15 patients.

A double-blind crossover comparative study of ondansetron and metoclopramide as single agents was carried out in 97 patients scheduled to receive cisplatin. The primary endpoint of the study was complete response (defined as no vomits) or near-complete response (less than two vomits) and control of acute vomiting. The primary endpoint was achieved in 46% and 29% of the patients, respectively, with ondansetron, 32 mg (8 mg intravenously, then 24 mg/24 hours intravenously), and in 16% and 26%, respectively, with metoclopramide. Acute nausea was less well controlled (complete control in 28% of patients) than acute emesis in this study and other trials conducted for similar indications.[13]

Two double-blind randomized placebo-controlled trials further demonstrated the efficacy of ondansetron in acute emesis. In these multicenter studies, ondansetron, 8 mg (either oral or parenteral), was more effective than metoclopramide in preventing acute emesis in patients receiving various combinations of emetogenic agents, including high doses of cyclophosphamide (2500 mg/m^2), doxorubicin (240 mg/m^2), epirubicin (240 mg/m^2) or 5-fluorouracil.[14, 15]

It is important to note that dexamethasone was not used with ondansetron in any of these early studies.

Efficacy over multiple-day chemotherapy cycles. Three early trials reported the use of ondansetron in 148 patients receiving 4–5 multiple-days of cisplatin chemotherapy (20–40 mg/m^2/day). In two of the studies, three daily intravenous doses of ondansetron, 0.15 mg/kg, were administered. The third study used three different doses of the antiemetic (0.015 mg/kg,

0.15 mg/kg or 0.3 mg/kg) given three times daily intravenously. 'No vomiting' response rates were between 21% and 35%.[16–18]

Efficacy in delayed CINV. Most early CINV studies reported poor control of delayed nausea and vomiting with ondansetron. In fact, the efficacy of ondansetron was no greater than that of conventional antiemetics in controlling delayed emesis. In a double-blind crossover study comparing ondansetron and dexamethasone, in which patients received intravenous non-platinum MEC (mostly comprising an anthracycline and/or cyclophosphamide and/or etoposide), delayed nausea (days 2–5) was significantly better controlled by dexamethasone alone than by ondansetron alone.[19]

Safety and tolerability. The overall safety of ondansetron is excellent; it is not associated with major side effects. Adverse events include headaches, diarrhea and constipation.

Extrapyramidal side effects are extremely rare. The FDA has recently restricted the intravenous dose to less than 16 mg because of prolongation of the QTc interval.

Tropisetron ([1H]-indol-3-carbonic-acid-tropinester hydrochloride) is licensed in Europe, Australia and a number of other countries for the treatment of CINV, but is not available in the USA.

Dosage. The recommended dose is 5 mg intravenously or orally. The infusion is administered shortly before chemotherapy.

Efficacy in acute CINV. A pilot study in 1987 determined that tropisetron had some effect over a wide dose range and that a single dose could reduce acute nausea and vomiting. Dose-finding studies demonstrated that tropisetron, 5 mg, provided total control of vomiting in up to 70% of patients during the first 24 hours after chemotherapy.

Tropisetron has been found to prevent acute nausea and vomiting induced by high doses of cisplatin. In a randomized crossover study of 20 patients receiving a mean cisplatin dose of 77.5 mg/m^2, tropisetron was significantly better ($p<0.001$) at controlling acute nausea and vomiting than a combination of metoclopramide and lorazepam.[20] Clinical experiences from various studies in patients receiving cisplatin, 50–120 mg/m², confirmed that tropisetron, 5 mg, administered intravenously or orally once daily, was more efficient in preventing acute CINV than metoclopramide, 4–7 mg/kg. When compared with antiemetic combinations based on high doses of metoclopramide, dexamethasone and lorazepam or diphenhydramine in patients receiving cisplatin-based chemotherapy, tropisetron was just as effective in preventing acute vomiting, but less effective in preventing acute nausea.

In patients undergoing bone marrow transplant receiving high-dose alkylating agents (cyclophosphamide, 7 g/m² in five 1-hour injections over 13 hours, or melphalan, 200 mg/m² in three intravenous boluses over 6 hours), tropisetron was more effective than alizapride in controlling acute vomiting. In the first 24 hours after treatment, the median number of vomiting episodes was five for patients treated with tropisetron, compared with nine in the alizapride group.[21]

Safety and tolerability. Headaches, constipation and diarrhea are the most frequent side effects. While these side effects are reported with similar frequency after metoclopramide treatment, the overall incidence of side effects appears to be greater for combinations of non-5-HT$_3$ agents.

Extrapyramidal side effects are extremely rare after tropisetron treatment.

Dolasetron (dolasetron mesylate) is a pseudopelletierine-derived 5-HT$_3$ antagonist. It is converted in vivo to its primary active metabolite, hydrodolasetron, which appears to be primarily responsible for its pharmacological action. Single oral or intravenous doses of dolasetron have shown efficacy in preventing acute CINV.

Dosage. The recommended dose is 5 mg intravenously or orally. The infusion is administered shortly before chemotherapy.

Efficacy in acute CINV. Intravenous doses of 1.8 mg/kg have been shown to attain complete control of vomiting in almost 50% of patients treated with cisplatin-based HEC and 60–80% of patients receiving MEC. Randomized trials have shown that intravenous dolasetron, 1.8 mg/kg, is equivalent to intravenous granisetron, 3 mg, or ondansetron, 32 mg, following HEC.[22, 23] Oral dolasetron, 200 mg, is equal to multiple doses of ondansetron given orally (three or four doses of 8 mg) after MEC.[24] Dolasetron, 1.8 mg/kg, has shown superiority over metoclopramide in preventing emesis by cisplatin-based HEC[25] or by MEC in high-risk subgroups.

Safety and tolerability. Dolasetron has a safety profile typical of this class of compounds, with headache and dizziness being the most common side effects. However, dolasetron is not recommended for CINV prophylaxis in Canada or the USA because it has been shown to prolong the QTc interval.

Palonosetron is a second-generation 5-HT$_3$ RA, approved for the prevention of acute and delayed CINV associated with MEC regimens and the prevention of acute CINV associated with HEC regimens. In fact, it is the first and only 5-HT$_3$ RA specifically indicated for the management of delayed CINV in patients receiving MEC.

Palonosetron is an isoquinolone hydrochloride that exists as a single isomer and is freely soluble in water. It has a 30-fold higher binding affinity for 5-HT$_3$ receptors and a longer plasma elimination half-life of approximately 40 hours than the first-generation 5-HT$_3$ RAs.

Palonosetron exhibits allosteric interactions and positive cooperativity with the 5-HT$_3$ receptor, characteristics not observed in the first-generation 5-HT$_3$ RAs (granisetron, ondansetron, tropisetron, dolasetron). The binding of palonosetron elicits receptor internalization, which results in prolonged inhibition of serotonin signaling. In addition, palonosetron inhibits cross-talk between serotonin/5-HT$_3$ and NK-1/substance P signaling pathways. These properties enable

33

palonosetron to maintain adequate 5-HT$_3$ receptor blockade even when it is no longer detectable in plasma, making it more effective and convenient than the first-generation RAs.

Dosage. The recommended dose is 0.25 mg intravenously or 0.5 mg orally. The oral formulation is not available in the USA.

Efficacy. A meta-analysis of 16 randomized clinical trials was performed comparing palonosetron to other 5-HT$_3$ RAs, involving 2896 patients who received palonosetron and 3187 patients randomized to other 5-HT$_3$ RAs. The meta-analysis showed that palonosetron was statistically superior to the other 5-HT$_3$ RAs in the acute, delayed and overall phases of CINV.[26] Essentially, when given without an NK-1 RA, palonosetron is more effective than other 5-HT$_3$ RAs in the management of CINV in patients receiving both MEC and HEC.

Safety and tolerability. Palonosetron's most common adverse effects are constipation, headache, diarrhea and dizziness.

Neurokinin-1 receptor antagonists

Aprepitant and fosaprepitant. Aprepitant is approved for the treatment of CINV in combination with a 5-HT$_3$ RA and dexamethasone. Fosaprepitant (a prodrug of aprepitant) is converted to aprepitant via phosphatase enzymes in the bloodstream. Fosaprepitant is an intravenous formulation that can be used in place of the oral dose of aprepitant on day 1. It may be advantageous in patients who cannot tolerate an oral formulation.

Dosage. Fosaprepitant, 115 mg intravenously, and oral aprepitant, 125 mg, are bioequivalent and interchangeable. Aprepitant is administered as three doses taken orally: 125 mg before chemotherapy on day 1, followed by 80 mg on days 2 and 3. Fosaprepitant is administered as a 150 mg intravenous injection before chemotherapy on day 1. A randomized phase III trial showed non-inferiority between these dosing regimens for the prevention of overall and delayed CINV.[27]

Efficacy in HEC. All clinical trials with aprepitant have shown very good clinical activity for patients receiving HEC.

In two phase III trials, a triple combination of aprepitant, ondansetron and dexamethasone was found to have significantly greater rates of complete response than ondansetron plus dexamethasone in patients receiving cisplatin-based HEC. Patients were randomized to receive standard therapy with intravenous ondansetron, 32 mg, and oral dexamethasone, 20 mg) on day 1 followed by dexamethasone, 8 mg twice daily on days 2–4, or the triple combination of oral aprepitant, 125 mg, intravenous ondansetron, 32 mg, and oral dexamethasone, 12 mg, on day 1 followed by aprepitant, 80 mg, and dexamethasone, 8 mg, once daily on days 2 and 3, followed by dexamethasone, 8 mg, on day 4. The two trials evaluated 523 and 521 patients for efficacy and 568 and 525 patients for safety, respectively. In a combined analysis of both studies, the complete response rates in the acute phase were 86% for the aprepitant group versus 73% in the active control group. The response rates for the delayed phase were 72% versus 51%, and 68% versus 48% for the overall 5-day period ($p<0.001$ for all time periods).[28] In both studies, aprepitant was well tolerated and the rates of adverse effects and discontinuations were comparable between the two treatment groups.

A separate randomized trial compared 3 days of aprepitant plus day-1 ondansetron and 4 days of dexamethasone to 4 days of ondansetron plus dexamethasone in 489 patients receiving multiple-day HEC. The complete response rates for overall, acute and delayed CINV were significantly greater in the aprepitant group. In the overall phase (days 1–5), 72% of those treated with aprepitant had a complete response compared with 61% of patients treated with 4 days of ondansetron plus dexamethasone.[29]

In a cisplatin-based HEC study, Kaplan–Meier curves of 'time to first emesis' showed that patients who received an antiemetic regimen containing aprepitant fared significantly better than patients who received only standard therapy ($p<0.001$); the treatment groups began to differ noticeably

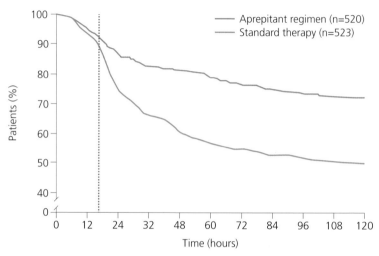

Figure 3.2 Percentage of patients receiving a first cycle of highly emetogenic chemotherapy who remain emesis free over time. The Kaplan–Meier curves show that a higher percentage of patients who received the aprepitant regimen remained emesis free than those receiving standard therapy ($p < 0.001$); the treatment groups began to differ noticeably about 16 hours after the administration of chemotherapy (dotted line). Reproduced with permission from Poli-Bigelli S et al.[30]

about 16 hours after the administration of chemotherapy (Figure 3.2).[30] Similar effects were observed with rolapitant (see Figure 3.4) and netupitant, suggesting a class effect of NK-1 RAs.

Efficacy in AC-based chemotherapy. Aprepitant has also proved effective in the management of CINV caused by anthracycline and cyclophosphamide (AC)-based chemotherapy. A study in women with breast cancer treated with AC-based chemotherapy showed that a three-drug antiemetic regimen with aprepitant had an overall complete response rate of 50%, compared with 42.5% achieved with a standard two-drug regimen without an NK-1 RA.[31] It is important to note that at the time of this study AC-based chemotherapy was classified as MEC, but has since been reclassified as HEC.

AC-based chemotherapy is monophasic, with both the 5-HT$_3$- and NK-1-mediated effects occurring within a few

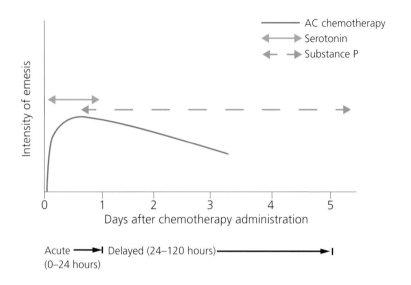

Figure 3.3 Monophasic pattern of emesis induced by anthracycline–cyclophosphamide (AC)-based chemotherapy, with both the serotonin (5-HT$_3$)- and neurokinin (NK)-1 (substance P)-mediated effects occurring within a few hours of chemotherapy, early in the acute phase.

hours after chemotherapy, early in the acute phase (Figure 3.3) In patients receiving AC-based treatment, aprepitant is effective at the beginning in the acute phase, as early as 6 hours after chemotherapy, compared with approximately 16 hours in the HEC study described above. This demonstrates that although the NK-1 RAs are associated fundamentally with delayed CINV, they also have a crucial function in the acute phase in both HEC and MEC.

Efficacy in MEC. Special consideration should be given to aprepitant in patients receiving non-AC-based MEC. A placebo-controlled randomized trial of 848 patients evaluated the efficacy of the same antiemetic regimen in a range of MEC regimens, including AC-, oxaliplatin- and carboplatin-based chemotherapies. Importantly, in this trial, more patients treated with aprepitant experienced no vomiting (76.2%) than those treated with the active control (62.1%).[32, 33] These data also

37

demonstrated that antiemetic regimens with aprepitant were active for non-AC-based chemotherapy regimens.

Safety and tolerability. Aprepitant and fosaprepitant may cause side effects, including serious allergic reactions such as hives, rash, itching and trouble breathing or swallowing. Severe skin reactions may occur rarely.

Inhibition of CYP3A4. Aprepitant and fosaprepitant should be used with caution in patients receiving concomitant medications that are primarily metabolized through CYP3A4, as inhibition of CYP3A4 by aprepitant or fosaprepitant could result in elevated plasma concentrations of the concurrent medications. When fosaprepitant is used concomitantly with another CYP3A4 inhibitor, aprepitant plasma concentrations could be elevated. When aprepitant is used concomitantly with medications that induce CYP3A4 activity, aprepitant plasma concentrations could be reduced, and this may result in decreased efficacy of aprepitant.

Chemotherapy agents known to be metabolized by CYP3A4 include docetaxel, paclitaxel, etoposide, irinotecan, ifosfamide, imatinib, vinorelbine, vinblastine and vincristine.

Infusion-site reactions have been shown to occur more often in patients receiving fosaprepitant (3.0%) than those receiving aprepitant (0.5%). The reported infusion-site reactions comprised erythema, pruritus, pain, induration and thrombophlebitis.

Rolapitant is a potent, selective, high-affinity, competitive NK-1 RA with an extended half-life of approximately 180 hours. It is licensed for the treatment of delayed CINV.

Dosage. Rolapitant is administered as a single oral dose of 180 mg before chemotherapy on day 1 of treatment. Positron emission tomography (PET) in healthy volunteers 120 hours after a single 180-mg oral dose of rolapitant demonstrated more than 90% NK-1 receptor occupancy in the subjects' brains.[34] This study indicates that a single dose of rolapitant may be sufficient to prevent CINV during the full risk period of 0 to 120 hours.

Efficacy in HEC. In a multicenter, double-blind, placebo-controlled, dose range-finding, phase II study, 454 patients being treated with HEC ($\geq$ 70 mg/m^2 cisplatin-based chemotherapy) were randomized to receive ondansetron plus dexamethasone and either placebo or 9, 22.5, 90 or 180 mg of rolapitant before chemotherapy on day 1 of each cycle. The rolapitant 180-mg group had a significantly greater complete response rate than the control group in the overall (62.5% vs 46.7%), acute (87.6% vs 66.7%) and delayed (63.6% vs 48.9%) phases.[35]

These findings were confirmed in two randomized double-blind active-controlled parallel-group phase III trials. Patients received oral rolapitant, 180 mg, or placebo before HEC administration. All patients received intravenous granisetron, 10 µg/kg, and oral dexamethasone, 20 mg, on day 1, and dexamethasone, 8 mg, on days 2–4. The primary endpoint was complete response (defined as no emesis or rescue medication) in the delayed phase (after 24 to 120 hours). Notably, both rolapitant HEC studies achieved the primary endpoint, and superiority of rolapitant was confirmed over the active control. The rolapitant-treated patients had significantly higher complete response rates than controls in the delayed phase (HEC-1: 72.7% vs 58.4% and HEC-2: 70.1% vs 61.9%; pooled studies: 71.4% vs 60.2%) (Figure 3.4).[36]

Efficacy in MEC. In a global, randomized, double-blind, active-controlled, parallel group, phase III study, 1322 MEC- and HEC-naive patients were randomized to receive oral rolapitant, 180 mg, or placebo approximately 30 minutes before administration of MEC. It is important to clarify that there were two cohorts receiving either AC-based (703 patients) or non-AC-based (629 patients) chemotherapy regimens, and at the time of protocol development AC-based regimens were classified as MEC; they are now classified as HEC. The primary endpoint of complete response consisting of no emesis or rescue treatment in the delayed phase (after 24 to 120 hours) was successfully achieved. Treatment with rolapitant resulted in a significantly higher complete response rate in the delayed phase

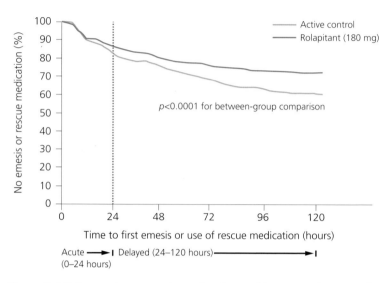

Figure 3.4 Estimates for proportions of patients without emesis or use of rescue medication (modified intention-to-treat population) from pooled HEC studies. The dotted line at 24 hours represents the division between the acute and delayed phases of chemotherapy-induced nausea and vomiting. Pooled HEC studies. Reproduced with permission from Rapoport BL et al. 2015.[36]

(71.3% vs 61.6%, $p<0.001$) than control treatment.[37] The trial demonstrated the advantage of adding an NK-1 RA to active control for the prevention of CINV in patients receiving both AC-based and non-AC-based MEC. A pre-specified exploratory logistic regression analysis, which adjusted for sex, region, age and use of AC-based chemotherapy confirmed the primary analysis. When analyzed by chemotherapy subgroups, treatment with rolapitant demonstrated significantly higher complete response rates than control treatment in the delayed phase in patients who received AC-based (66.9% vs 59.5%; $p=0.05$) and non-AC-based (76.1% vs 63.8%; $p\leq0.001$) MEC.[37] It is important to highlight that the randomization of the AC and non-AC groups was done prospectively with a prespecified endpoint. These data clearly show that rolapitant is active in CINV prophylaxis in patients receiving non-AC-based MEC.

Safety and tolerability. The most common adverse reactions (≥ 5%) are neutropenia, hiccups, decreased appetite and dizziness. The incidence of these side effects was similar to those reported in the control arm in the rolapitant registration studies.

Rolapitant is not an inhibitor or inducer of CYP3A4, so it is unlikely to have drug–drug interactions with drugs metabolized by CYP3A4, such as those given to patients undergoing chemotherapy. This means that dose adjustments for concomitant anticancer agents administered with other NK-1 RAs, which could result in a potential loss of efficiency and inferior outcome, may not be required with rolapitant.

Netupitant and NEPA. Netupitant is available in combination with oral palonosetron (NEPA) for the management and prophylaxis of CINV. NEPA consists of a fixed-dose of netupitant (a potent and selective NK-1 RA) in combination with a fixed dose of palonosetron, thereby targeting two antiemetic pathways.

Dosage. One NEPA capsule comprises netupitant, 300 mg, and palonosetron, 0.5 mg, and should be administered approximately 1 hour before the start of chemotherapy.

Efficacy. NEPA has been studied in phase II and III clinical trials for the prevention of CINV in patients treated with MEC and HEC. These clinical trials revealed that NEPA significantly enhanced the prophylaxis of CINV compared with the administration of palonosetron alone. NEPA was associated with a significant improvement in delayed CINV (24–120 hours) and the overall CINV period (0–120 hours). This effect continued over multiple cycles of treatment.

Efficacy in HEC. A randomized, double-blind, parallel-group trial compared three different formulations of NEPA – oral netupitant, 100, 200 or 300 mg, plus oral palonsetron, 0.5 mg – with palonosetron, 0.5 mg, alone in 694 chemotherapy-naive patients being treated with cisplatin-based HEC. Treatment was given before chemotherapy on day 1. An additional comparator control arm was used, comprising standard 3-day oral aprepitant, 125 mg on day 1 followed by 80 mg on days 2 and 3, and intravenous ondansetron, 32 mg. Patients in all treatment arms were given oral dexamethasone on days 1–4. The primary efficacy endpoint was complete response for the overall phase (0–120 hours). All the NEPA arms of the study were significantly superior for overall complete response rates compared with palonosetron alone. The 300-mg NEPA dose showed a numerical improvement over the lower doses. In addition, no significant difference was detected in the overall complete response between the NEPA and aprepitant treatment arms.[38]

NEPA had a low incidence of adverse events in all treatment groups.

Efficacy in AC-based chemotherapy. A phase III, multinational, randomized, double-blind, parallel-group study, compared the efficacy and safety of a single oral dose of NEPA (netupitant, 300 mg, and palonosetron, 0.5 mg) with a palonosetron, 0.5 mg, alone in 1455 chemotherapy-naive patients receiving repeated cycles of anthracycline-based chemotherapy. All patients in the NEPA arm received oral dexamethasone, 12 mg, while those in the palonosetron arm were given dexamethasone, 20 mg, on the first day of each cycle. Most patients were Caucasian women undergoing treatment for breast cancer. The primary endpoint of the trial was complete response in the delayed phase (25–120 hours). NEPA showed superior complete response rates in the delayed, acute and overall phases. NEPA was also better than palonosetron during the delayed and overall phases for complete protection, defined as no emesis and no significant nausea.[39]

The authors concluded that NEPA was superior to palonosetron in preventing CINV in patients with breast cancer receiving MEC. Treatment with NEPA was well tolerated, and there was no evidence of any cardiac safety concerns for NEPA or palonosetron. The frequency of headaches was 3.3% and constipation 2.1%.[39]

Safety and tolerability. Most common adverse reactions (incidence ≥ 3% and greater than palonosetron) are headache, asthenia, dyspepsia, fatigue, constipation and erythema. Inhibition of CYP3A4 by netupitant can result in increased plasma concentrations of the concomitant drug that can last at least 4 days and may last longer after single-dose administration of NEPA. Concurrent usage with CYP3A4 inducers such as rifampicin (rifampin) may result in decreased plasma concentrations of netupitant.

Corticosteroids

Although the mechanism of action of corticosteroids in CINV is unknown, they are effective agents in the management of acute and delayed CINV both as monotherapy and in combination with other agents (either with a 5-HT$_3$ RA alone or as part of a triple-drug regimen with an NK-1 RA). They have remained valuable agents even since the development of NK-1 RAs and the first second-generation 5-HT$_3$ RA, palonosetron, and remain the backbone of most CINV prophylactic regimens.

Dexamethasone is the most broadly used corticosteroid in the management of CINV. Although dexamethasone is not approved as an antiemetic, it plays a significant role in the prophylaxis of acute and delayed CINV, and is an essential part of almost all antiemetic regimens in clinical practice.

Safety and tolerability. Corticosteroids used in CINV as either monotherapy or in combination with other agents are very well tolerated. The most common side effects are transient elevations in glucose, insomnia, anxiety and gastric upset.[40, 41] In most settings, the duration of therapy with a corticosteroid is short and side effects can be managed, and the benefits are considered to offset any adverse effects. Uncommonly, these agents can decompensate diabetes, cause psychosis, or reactivate an ulcer. Importantly, when combined with aprepitant, the dose of dexamethasone should be reduced, as dexamethasone is a sensitive substrate of the cytochrome P450 [CYP] 3A4 enzyme.

Dopamine receptor antagonists

The CTZ contains D2, 5-HT_3 and NK-1 neuroreceptors, and it is the site of action for dopamine receptor antagonists. Situated outside the blood–brain barrier, it is exposed to toxins such as chemotherapy in the bloodstream and cerebral spinal fluid, and dopamine RAs work in this neural pathway to trigger vomiting. The prototype agent in this category is metoclopramide. Others include domperidone and butyrophenones like droperidol and haloperidol. Chlorpromazine and prochlorperazine have also been used.

Dosage. The maximum advocated dose of metoclopramide in adults has been restricted to 30 mg/day.

Safety and tolerability. Metoclopramide has the tendency to cause extrapyramidal side effects, including acute dystonic reactions, akathisia and sedation, which limit its use. The European Medicines Agency has restricted metoclopramide to short-term use (up to 5 days) to lessen the potential of neurological side effects such as extrapyramidal disorders.

Olanzapine

Olanzapine is an antipsychotic thiobenzodiazepine agent with antiemetic properties as a result of its ability to target dopaminergic (D_1, D_2, D_3, D_4), serotonergic (5-HT_{2A}, 5-HT_{2C}, 5-HT_3, 5-HT_6), adrenergic ($\alpha\text{-}1$), histaminergic (H_1) and muscarinic (m_1, m_2, m_3, m_4) receptors. This ability to target multiple key receptors with one medication gives olanzapine an advantage over combination CINV treatments.

Dosage of olanzapine for CINV prophylaxis and treatment is 5–10 mg/day for 4 days. It is available as a generic.

Efficacy in HEC and MEC. Phase I and II clinical studies established that olanzapine can improve complete responses for delayed CINV in patients taking HEC and MEC, as well as improve the quality of life of patients with cancer during chemotherapy.[42-44]

In a phase III trial, chemotherapy-naive patients undergoing HEC regimens of cisplatin, 70 mg/m^2, or cyclophosphamide, 500 mg/m^2 and doxorubicin, 50 mg/m^2 were randomized to receive either oral olanzapine, 10 mg, intravenous palonosetron, 0.25 mg, and intravenous dexamethasone, 20 mg, on day 1 followed by olanzapine, 10 mg, on days 2–4 after chemotherapy or oral aprepitant, 125 mg, intravenous palonosetron, 0.25 mg, and intravenous dexamethasone, 12 mg, on day 1 followed by oral aprepitant, 80 mg, and oral dexamethasone, 4 mg, twice daily on days 2–4. In the olanzapine group, no vomiting occurred in either the olanzapine or aprepitant group and no rescue was needed in 97% vs 87% of patients during the acute phase in the olanazapine and aprepitant groups, respectively, in 77% vs 73% during the delayed phase, and in 77% vs 73% overall.[45]

No nausea was experienced in 87% vs 87% in the acute phase, 69% vs 28% during the delayed phase, and 69% vs 38% overall in the olanzapine and aprepitant groups, respectively.

Efficacy in breakthrough CINV was also investigated in a phase III trial in which patients were randomized to receive oral olanzapine, 10 mg three times daily for 3 days, or oral metoclopramide, 10 mg three times daily for 3 days, then monitored for 72 hours. Patients were treated with HEC of either cisplatin, 70 mg/m^2, or cyclophosphamide, 600 mg/m^2, and doxorubicin, 50 mg/m^2, with prophylactic antiemetics of intravenous dexamethasone, 12 mg, intravenous palonosetron, 0.25 mg, and intravenous fosaprepitant, 150 mg, on day 1 and then oral dexamethasone, 8 mg, on days 2–4. No vomiting occurred in 70% vs 31% of patients in the olanzapine and metoclopramide groups, respectively, and 68% vs 23% of patients reported no nausea.[46]

Safety and tolerability. Olanzapine has been associated with only mild sedation when used for the prevention of CINV in clinical trials.

Ginger

Some studies have evaluated ginger's potential in preventing chemotherapy-induced nausea. Two studies showed that ginger supplementation at daily doses of 0.5, 1.0 or 1.5 g significantly reduced the severity of acute chemotherapy-induced nausea compared with placebo in patients receiving standard 5-HT$_3$ RA prophylaxis in combination with dexamethasone. However, more severe delayed nausea was reported by patients than acute nausea. Importantly, a significant benefit of ginger in the delayed phase was not seen.[47, 48]

Cannabinoids

Cannabinoids are molecules present in the cannabis plant. They bind to cannabinoid receptors, and pharmacologically their effects include appetite stimulation and analgesia. Cannabinoids also inhibit multiple neurotransmitter systems involved in nausea and vomiting reflexes.

Dronabinol and nabilone are two oral formulations approved in several countries for use in CINV that is refractory to conventional antiemetic therapy.[49, 50] To improve antiemetic therapy across the entire spectrum of CINV requires the use of agents with different mechanisms of action. Cannabinoids may be effective in the management of nausea, which remains the greatest unmet medical need in medical research. However, the side effects of these agents may have delayed their use in clinical practice.

The use of marijuana remains legally and therapeutically controversial. In the future, new and less toxic formulations of cannabinoids may play a significant role in CINV management. Currently, cannabinoids are not recommended for management of CINV and are not part of any major clinical antiemetic guidelines.

Key points – antiemetic agents

- Serotonin (5-HT$_3$) receptor antagonists (RAs) (ondansetron, granisetron, tropisetron, dolasetron and palonosetron) have their main antiemetic effect during the acute CINV phase.
- Neurokinin (NK)-1 receptor antagonists (aprepitant, fosaprepitant, rolapitant and netupitant) have their main antiemetic effect during the delayed CINV phase.
- Corticosteroids (dexamethasone in particular) have a significant role in the prophylaxis of acute and delayed CINV, and are an essential part of almost all antiemetic regimens in clinical practice.
- A combination of a triple antiemetic regimen of a 5-HT$_3$ RA, an NK-1 RA and a corticosteroid is very effective in antiemetic prophylaxis for patients receiving cispatin, AC (anthracycline and cyclophosphamide)-based and highly emetogenic chemotherapy (HEC) regimens.
- Recent data have shown that a combination of a triple antiemetic regimen of a 5-HT$_3$ RA, an NK-1 RA and a corticosteroid is very effective in the prophylaxis of moderately emetogenic chmeotherapy (MEC) regimens, in particular carboplatin-based treatment.
- 5-HT$_3$ RAs, NK-1 RAs and corticosteroids are not very effective in the prophylaxis of chemotherapy-induced nausea. Nausea control remains a challenge in the management of CINV.

Key references

1. Tavorath R, Hesketh P. Drug treatment of chemotherapy-induced delayed emesis. *Drugs* 2013;52:639–48.

2. Martin M. The severity and pattern of emesis following different cytotoxic agents. *Oncology* 1996;53:26–31.

3. Navari RM, Kaplan HG, Gralla RJ et al. Efficacy and safety of granisetron, a selective 5-hydroxytryptamine-3 receptor antagonist, in the prevention of nausea and vomiting induced by high-dose cisplatin. *J Clin Oncol* 1994;12:2204–10.

4. Bleiberg HH, Spielmann M, Falkson G, Romain D. Antiemetic treatment with oral granisetron in patients receiving moderately emetogenic chemotherapy: a dose-ranging study. *Clin Ther* 1995;17:38–51.

5. Cupissol DR, Serron B, Canbel M. The efficacy of granisetron as a prophylactic anti-emetic and intervention agent in high-dose cisplatin-induced emesis. *Eur J Cancer* 1990;26(Suppl 1):S23–7.

6. Roila F, Tonato M, Basurto C et al. Protection from nausea and vomiting in cisplatin-treated patients: high-dose metoclopramide combined with methylprednisolone versus metoclopramide combined with dexamethasone and diphenhydramine: a study of the Italian Oncology Group for Clinical Research. *J Clin Oncol* 1989;7:1693–700.

7. Marty M. A comparative study of the use of granisetron, a selective 5-HT3 antagonist, versus a standard anti-emetic regimen of chlorpromazine plus dexamethasone in the treatment of cytostatic-induced emesis. The Granisetron Study Group. *Eur J Cancer* 1990;26(Suppl 1):S28–32.

8. Blijham GH; Granisetron Study Group. Doses granisetron remain effective over multiple cycles? *Eur J Cancer* 1992;28A(Suppl 1):S17–21.

9. Diehl V. Fractionated chemotherapy – granisetron or conventional antiemetics? The Granisetron Study Group. *Eur J Cancer* 1992;28A(Suppl 1):S21–8.

10. Boccia RV, Gordon LN, Clark G et al. Efficacy and tolerability of transdermal granisetron for the control of chemotherapy-induced nausea and vomiting associated with moderately and highly emetogenic multiple-day chemotherapy: a randomized, double-blind, phase III study. *Support Care Cancer* 2011;19:1609–17.

11. Schnadig ID, Agajanian R, Dakhil SR et al. Phase III study of APF530 versus ondansetron with a neurokinin 1 antagonist + corticosteroid in preventing highly emetogenic chemotherapy-induced nausea and vomiting: MAGIC trial. 2015 Breast Cancer Symposium. *J Clin Oncol* 2015;33(suppl 28S): abstr 68.

12. Raftopoulos H, Boccia R, Cooper W et al. Slow-release granisetron (APF530) versus palonosetron for chemotherapy-induced nausea/vomiting: analysis by American Society of Clinical Oncology emetogenicity criteria. *Future Oncol* 2015;11:2541–51.

13. Marty M, Pouillart P, Scholl S et al. Comparison of the 5-hydroxytryptamine 3 (serotonin) antagonist ondansetron (GR 38032F) with high-dose metoclopramide in the control of cisplatin-induced emesis. *N Engl J Med* 1990;322:816–21.

14. Kaasa S, Kvaløy S, Dicato MA et al. A comparison of ondansetron with metoclopramide in the prophylaxis of chemotherapy-induced nausea and vomiting: a randomized, double-blind study. International Emesis Study Group. *Eur J Cancer* 1990;26:311–14.

15. Bonneterre J, Chevallier B, Metz R et al. A randomized double-blind comparison of ondansetron and metoclopramide in the prophylaxis of emesis induced by cyclophosphamide, fluorouracil, and doxorubicin or epirubicin chemotherapy. *J Clin Oncol* 1990;8:1063–9.

16. Einhorn LH, Nagy C, Werner K, Finn AL. Ondansetron: a new antiemetic for patients receiving cisplatin chemotherapy. *J Clin Oncol* 1990;8:731–5.

17. Hainsworth JD, Omura GA, Khojasteh A et al. Ondansetron (GR 38032F): a novel antiemetic effective in patients receiving a multiple-day regimen of cisplatin chemotherapy. *Am J Clin Oncol* 1991;14:336–40.

18. Sledge GW Jr, Einhorn L, Nagy C, House K. Phase III double-blind comparison of intravenous ondansetron and metoclopramide as antiemetic therapy for patients receiving multiple-day cisplatin-based chemotherapy. *Cancer* 1992;70:2524–8.

19. Jones AL, Hill AS, Soukop M et al. Comparison of dexamethasone and ondansetron in the prophylaxis of emesis induced by moderately emetogenic chemotherapy. *Lancet* 1991;338:483–7.

20. Dogliotti L, Antonacci RA, Pazè E et al. Three years' experience with tropisetron in the control of nausea and vomiting in cisplatin-treated patients. *Drugs* 1992;43(Suppl 3): 6–10.

21. De Nigris A, Paladini G, Giosa F et al. Tropisetron (Navoban) compared with alizapride in the control of emesis induced by cyclophosphamide-containing regimens. *Eur J Cancer* 1994;30A:1902–3.

22. Audhuy B, Cappelaere P, Martin M et al. A double-blind, randomised comparison of the anti-emetic efficacy of two intravenous doses of dolasetron mesilate and granisetron in patients receiving high dose cisplatin chemotherapy. *Eur J Cancer* 1996;32A:807–13.

23. Hesketh P, Navari R, Grote T et al. Double-blind, randomized comparison of the antiemetic efficacy of intravenous dolasetron mesylate and intravenous ondansetron in the prevention of acute cisplatin-induced emesis in patients with cancer. Dolasetron Comparative Chemotherapy-induced Emesis Prevention Group. *J Clin Oncol* 1996;14:2242–9.

24. Lofters WS, Pater JL, Zee B et al. Phase III double-blind comparison of dolasetron mesylate and ondansetron and an evaluation of the additive role of dexamethasone in the prevention of acute and delayed nausea and vomiting due to moderately emetogenic chemotherapy. *J Clin Oncol* 1997;15:2966–73.

25. Chevallier B, Cappelaere P, Splinter T et al. A double-blind, multicentre comparison of intravenous dolasetron mesilate and metoclopramide in the prevention of nausea and vomiting in cancer patients receiving high-dose cisplatin chemotherapy. *Support Care Cancer* 1997;5:22–30.

26. Popovic M, Warr DG, Deangelis C et al. Efficacy and safety of palonosetron for the prophylaxis of chemotherapy-induced nausea and vomiting (CINV): a systematic review and meta-analysis of randomized controlled trials. *Support Care Cancer* 2014;22:1685–97.

27. Grunberg S, Chua D, Maru A et al. Single-dose fosaprepitant for the prevention of chemotherapy-induced nausea and vomiting associated with cisplatin therapy: randomized, double-blind study protocol--EASE. *J Clin Oncol* 2011;29:1495–501.

28. Hesketh PJ, Grunberg SM, Herrstedt J et al. Combined data from two phase III trials of the NK1 antagonist aprepitant plus a 5HT3 antagonist and a corticosteroid for prevention of chemotherapy-induced nausea and vomiting: effect of gender on treatment response. *Support Care Cancer* 2006;14:354–60.

29. Schmoll HJ, Aapro MS, Poli-Bigelli S et al. Comparison of an aprepitant regimen with a multiple-day ondansetron regimen, both with dexamethasone, for antiemetic efficacy in high-dose cisplatin treatment. *Ann Oncol* 2006;17:1000–6.

30. Poli-Bigelli S, Rodrigues-Pereira J, Carides AD et al.; Aprepitant Protocol 054 Study Group. Addition of the neurokinin 1 receptor antagonist aprepitant to standard antiemetic therapy improves control of chemotherapy-induced nausea and vomiting. Results from a randomized, double-blind, placebo-controlled trial in Latin America. *Cancer* 2003;97:3090–8.

31. Warr DG, Hesketh PJ, Gralla RJ et al. Efficacy and tolerability of aprepitant for the prevention of chemotherapy-induced nausea and vomiting in patients with breast cancer after moderately emetogenic chemotherapy. *J Clin Oncol* 2005;23:2822–30.

32. Rapoport BL, Jordan K, Boice JA et al. Aprepitant for the prevention of chemotherapy-induced nausea and vomiting associated with a broad range of moderately emetogenic chemotherapies and tumor types: a randomized, double-blind study. *Support Care Cancer* 2010;18:423–31.

33. Rapoport BL. Efficacy of a triple antiemetic regimen with aprepitant for the prevention of chemotherapy-induced nausea and vomiting: effects of gender, age, and region. *Curr Med Res Opin* 2014;30:1875–81.

34. Poma, A, Christensen, J, Davis J et al. Phase 1 positron emission tomography (PET) study of the receptor occupancy of rolapitant, a novel NK-1 receptor antagonist. *J Clin Oncol* 2014;32(abstr e20690).

35. Rapoport B, Chua D, Poma A et al. Study of rolapitant, a novel, long-acting, NK-1 receptor antagonist, for the prevention of chemotherapy-induced nausea and vomiting (CINV) due to highly emetogenic chemotherapy (HEC). *Support Care Cancer* 2015;23:3281–8.

36. Rapoport BL, Chasen MR, Gridelli C. Safety and efficacy of rolapitant for prevention of chemotherapy-induced nausea and vomiting after administration of cisplatin-based highly emetogenic chemotherapy in patients with cancer: two randomised, active-controlled, double-blind, phase 3 trials. *Lancet Oncol* 2015;16:1079–89.

37. Schwartzberg LS, Modiano MR, Rapoport BL et al. Safety and efficacy of rolapitant for prevention of chemotherapy-induced nausea and vomiting after administration of moderately emetogenic chemotherapy or anthracycline and cyclophosphamide regimens in patients with cancer: a randomised, active-controlled, double-blind, phase 3 trial. *Lancet Oncol* 2015;16:1071–8.

38. Hesketh PJ, Rossi G, Rizzi G et al. Efficacy and safety of NEPA, an oral combination of netupitant and palonosetron, for prevention of chemotherapy-induced nausea and vomiting following highly emetogenic chemotherapy: a randomized dose-ranging pivotal study. *Ann Oncol* 2014;25:1340–6.

39. Aapro M, Rugo H, Rossi G et al. A randomized phase III study evaluating the efficacy and safety of NEPA, a fixed-dose combination of netupitant and palonosetron, for prevention of chemotherapy-induced nausea and vomiting following moderately emetogenic chemotherapy. *Ann Oncol* 2014;25:1328–33.

40. Ioannidis JP, Hesketh PJ, Lau J. Contribution of dexamethasone to control of chemotherapy-induced nausea and vomiting: a meta-analysis of randomized evidence. *J Clin Oncol* 2000;18:3409–22.

41. Vardy J, Chiew KS, Galica J et al. Side effects associated with the use of dexamethasone for prophylaxis of delayed emesis after moderately emetogenic chemotherapy. *Br J Cancer* 2006;94:1011–15.

42. Chow R, Chiu L, Navari R et al. Efficacy and safety of olanzapine for the prophylaxis of chemotherapy-induced nausea and vomiting (CINV) as reported in phase I and II studies: a systematic review. *Support Care Cancer* 2016;24:1001–8.

43. Navari RM, Einhorn LH, Passik SD et al. A phase II trial of olanzapine for the prevention of chemotherapy-induced nausea and vomiting: a Hoosier Oncology Group study. *Support Care Cancer* 2005;13:529–34.

44. Passik SD, Navari RM, Jung SH et al. A phase I trial of olanzapine (Zyprexa) for the prevention of delayed emesis in cancer patients: a Hoosier Oncology Group study. *Cancer Invest* 2004;22:383–8.

45. Navari RM, Gray SE, Kerr AC. Olanzapine versus aprepitant for the prevention of chemotherapy-induced nausea and vomiting: a randomized phase III trial. *J Support Oncol* 2011;9:188–95.

46. Navari RM, Nagy CK, Gray SE. The use of olanzapine versus metoclopramide for the treatment of breakthrough chemotherapy-induced nausea and vomiting in patients receiving highly emetogenic chemotherapy. *Support Care Cancer* 2013;21:1655–63.

47. Ryan JL, Heckler CE, Roscoe JA et al. Ginger (Zingiber officinale) reduces acute chemotherapy-induced nausea: a URCC CCOP study of 576 patients. *Support Care Cancer* 2012;20:1479–89.

48. Panahi Y, Saadat A, Sahebkar A et al. Effect of ginger on acute and delayed chemotherapy-induced nausea and vomiting: a pilot, randomized, open-label clinical trial. *Integr Cancer Ther* 2012;11:204–11.

49. Borgelt LM, Franson KL, Nussbaum AM, Wang GS. The pharmacologic and clinical effects of medical cannabis. *Pharmacotherapy* 2013;33:195–209.

50. Todaro B. Cannabinoids in the treatment of chemotherapy-induced nausea and vomiting. *J Natl Compr Canc Netw* 2012;10:487–92.

Further reading

Billio A, Morello E, Clarke MJ. Serotonin receptor antagonists for highly emetogenic chemotherapy in adults. *Cochrane Database Syst Rev* 2010;20(1):CD006272.

Chiu L, Chow R, Popovic M et al. Efficacy of olanzapine for the prophylaxis and rescue of chemotherapy-induced nausea and vomiting (CINV): a systematic review and meta-analysis. *Support Care Cancer* 2016;Jan 15 [Epub ahead of print].

Jordan K, Jahn F, Aapro M. Recent developments in the prevention of chemotherapy-induced nausea and vomiting (CINV): a comprehensive review. *Ann Oncol* 2015;26:1081–90.

Lorusso V, Karthaus M, Aapro M. Review of oral fixed-dose combination netupitant and palonosetron (NEPA) for the treatment of chemotherapy-induced nausea and vomiting. *Future Oncol* 2015;11:565–77.

Navari RM. Rolapitant for the treatment of chemotherapy-induced nausea and vomiting. *Expert Rev Anticancer Ther* 2015;15:1127–33.

Navari RM. Management of chemotherapy-induced nausea and vomiting: focus on newer agents and new uses for older agents. *Drugs* 2013;73:249–62.

It is essential that oncologists and oncology practitioners take significant time and effort to prepare patients adequately for their first course of chemotherapy. Clinicians have a wide variety of antiemetics to choose from for the prevention of chemotherapy-induced nausea and vomiting (CINV), and patients should receive the most effective antiemetic agents available.

Outcomes are improved by following the recommendations of national or international guidelines for CINV. Both the Multinational Association for Supportive Care in Cancer/European Society for Medical Oncology (MASCC/ESMO) and American Society of Clinical Oncology (ASCO) guidelines concur that the primary goal of CINV therapy is not to manage nausea and vomiting but to prevent these symptoms from happening in the first place.[1-4] All of the guidance for managing CINV in this book adheres to these international guidelines.[1-5]

If antiemetic therapy is used correctly, CINV can be prevented in up to 70–75% of patients receiving highly emetogenic chemotherapy (HEC) and up to 80% receiving moderately emetogenic chemotherapy (MEC).[5]

Management principles

Patients should be individually evaluated for their specific risk factors (see Table 2.2, page 18), as well as the level of anxiety present before the first course of treatment (see page 72). If the patient has a high level of anxiety before the first course of chemotherapy, serious consideration should be given to adding an antianxiety agent to the antiemetic regimen. To select the optimal antiemetic regimen, the emetogenic potential of the individual chemotherapy agents (Table 4.1) and overall emetogenicity of the chemotherapy regimen (Table 4.2) must be taken into consideration, according to the well-established antiemetic guidelines described above.[1-4]

TABLE 4.1

The emetogenic potential of individual chemotherapy agents

Emetogenic potential*	Agent (intravenous)	Agent (oral)
High Emesis in nearly all patients (> 90%)	*Alkylating agents* • Carmustine • Chlormethine* • Cisplatin • Cyclophosphamide ≥ 1500 mg/m^2 • Dacarbazine • Melphalan > 100 mg/m^2 • Streptozotocin *Antitumor antibiotics* • Dactinomycin[†]	*Alkylating agents* • Altretamine (Hexamethylmelamine) • Procarbazine
Moderate Emesis in 30–90% of patients	*Alkylating agents* • Bendamustine • Carboplatin • Cyclophosphamide < 1500 mg/m^2 • Ifosfamide • Oxaliplatin *Antimetabolites* • Clofarabine • Cytarabine > 1000 mg/m^2 *Antitumor antibiotics (anthracyclines)* • Daunorubicin[‡] • Doxorubicin[‡] • Epirubicin[‡] • Idrarubicin[‡]	*Alklyating agents* • Cyclophosphamide • Temozolomide *Plant alkaloids* • Vinorelbine *Tyrosine kinase inhibitors* • Imatinib

CONTINUED

TABLE 4.1 *CONTINUED*

Moderate Emesis in 30–90% of patients	*Demethylation agents* • Azacitidine *Monoclonal antibodies* • Alemtuzumab *Plant alkaloids* • Irinotecan	
Low Emesis in 10–30% of patients	*Antimetabolites* • 5-Fluorouracil • Cytarabine $\leq$ 1000 mg/m^2 • Gemcitabine • Methotrexate • Pemetrexed *Antitumor antibiotics* • Doxorubicin HCl liposome injection • Mitomycin • Mitoxantrone *Monoclonal antibodies* • Catumaxomab • Cetuximab[§] • Panitumumab • Trastuzumab *Plant alkaloids* • Cabazitaxel[†] • Docetaxel • Etoposide • Paclitaxel • Topotecan *Other agents* • Bortezomib • Ixabepilone • Temsirolimus	*Antimetabolites* • Capecitabine • Fludarabine • Tegafur with uracil *Immunomodulatory drugs* • Lenalidomide • Thalidomide *Plant alkaloids* • Etoposide *mTor inhibitors* • Everolimus *Tyrosine kinase inhibitors* • Lapatinib • Sunitinib

CONTINUED

55

TABLE 4.1 *CONTINUED*

Emetogenic potential*	Agent (intravenous)	Agent (oral)
Minimal Emesis in < 10% of patients	*Alkylating agents* • Busulfan *Antimetabolites* • Cladribine (2-Chlorodeoxyadenosine) • Fludarabine • Pralatrexate[†] *Antitumor antibiotics* • Bleomycin *Monoclonal antibodies* • Bevacizumab • Rituximab[†] *Plant alkaloids* • Vinblastine • Vincristine • Vinorelbine	*Alkylating agents* • Chlorambucil • L-Phenylalanine mustard *Antimetabolites* • 6-Thioguanine • Hyroxyurea • Methotrexate *Tyrosine kinase inhibitors* • Erlotinib • Gefitinib • Sorafenib

*Widely known as mechlorethamine in the USA (although not the USAN). [†]Listed in the ASCO antiemetic guidelines only. [‡]When combined with cyclophosphamide this anthracycline is now considered to be highly emetogenic chemotherapy. [§]Listed as having 'minimal' emetogenicity in the ASCO antiemetic guidelines.CINV, chemotherapy-induced nausea and vomiting.

Adapted from Gralla RJ et al. 2013, and Basch E et al. 2011 (MASCC/ESMO and ASCO Antiemetic Guidelines).[1,3]

Antiemetic therapy should be started before chemotherapy is administered on day 1 and continued through the acute and delayed phase for as long as the chemotherapy is emetic (usually 2–3 days). The route of delivery will depend on what the patient is best able to tolerate. In general, antiemetics given either orally or intravenously in appropriate doses have equivalent efficacy. If CINV can be prevented after the first course of chemotherapy, it is likely that subsequent courses of

TABLE 4.2

Guideline-directed antiemetic regimens according to type of chemotherapy*

Risk level	Chemotherapy	Recommended antiemetic regimen
High (> 90%)	Cisplatin and other HEC	*Acute CINV:* Day 1: 5-HT$_3$ RA + DEX + NK-1 RA[†] *Delayed CINV:* Days 2–3: DEX + NK-1 RA[‡]; day 4: DEX
	AC	*Acute CINV:* Day 1: 5-HT$_3$ RA + DEX + NK-1 RA[§] *Delayed CINV:* Days 2–3: NK-1 RA[‡]
Moderate (30–90%)	Non-AC MEC	*Acute CINV:* Day 1: 5-HT$_3$ RA[**] + DEX *Delayed CINV:* Days 2–3: DEX
	Carboplatin-based MEC	*Acute CINV:* Day 1: 5-HT$_3$ RA + DEX + NK-1 RA *Delayed CINV:* Days 2–3: NK-1 RA[‡] (+ DEX – see page 62)
Low (10–30%)		*Acute CINV:* Day 1: DEX or 5-HT$_3$ RA or dopamine RA *Delayed CINV:* Days 2–3: no routine prophylaxis
Minimal (< 10%)		*Acute CINV:* Day 1: no routine prophylaxis *Delayed CINV:* Days 2–3: no routine prophylaxis

*See Table 4.1 for emetogenic potential of individual chemotherapy agents. [†]NK-1 RAs include aprepitant, fosaprepitant, netupitant (in combination with palonosetron [NEPA]) and rolapitant. [‡]Only if aprepitant is used on day 1. If fosaprepitant is used, then dexamethasone only should be given for delayed CINV. [§]If the NK-1 RA is not available for AC chemotherapy, palonosetron is the preferred 5-HT$_3$ RA. [**]Palonosetron is the preferred 5-HT$_3$ RA for this indication.

5-HT$_3$, 5-hydroxytryptamine 3; AC, anthracycline and cyclophosphamide; DEX, dexamethasone; HEC, highly emetogenic chemotherapy; MEC, moderately emetogenic chemotherapy; NK-1, neurokinin-1; RA, receptor antagonist.

Adapted from Gralla RJ et al. 2013; Hesketh PJ et al. 2016; and Basch E et al. 2011 (MASCC/ESMO and ASCO Antiemetic Guidelines).[1–3] chemotherapy will be well tolerated and breakthrough, refractory and anticipatory CINV will be minimized.

Highly emetogenic chemotherapy

Prophylactic control of acute and delayed CINV that occurs as a result of cisplatin- or anthracycline and cyclophosphamide (AC)-based chemotherapy or other highly emetogenic chemotherapy (HEC) requires an initial three-drug regimen, administered before chemotherapy starts on day 1 of treatment (Figures 4.1 and 4.2). This should include a 5-HT$_3$ receptor

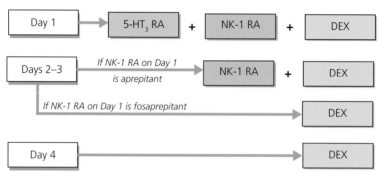

Figure 4.1 Guideline-directed treatment for acute and delayed CINV for patients receiving cisplatin- or other highly emetogenic chemotherapy.

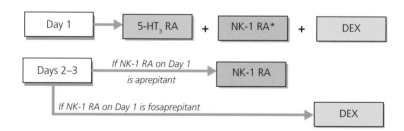

Figure 4.2 Guideline-directed treatment for acute and delayed CINV for patients receiving anthracycline and cyclophosphamide (AC)-based chemotherapy. *If the NK-1 RA is not available for day 1 prophylaxis, palonosetron is the preferred 5-HT$_3$ RA. Note that AC chemotherapy was recently reclassified from moderately emetogenic to highly emetogenic.

antagonist (RA) (granisetron, ondansetron, tropisetron, dolasetron or palonosetron; see pages 25–34), dexamethasone (see page 43) and a neurokinin (NK)-1 RA (aprepitant, fosaprepitant, rolapitant or netupitant/NEPA; see pages 34–43). The recommended doses for these agents are shown in Table 4.3.

Women with breast cancer receiving AC chemotherapy have a particularly high risk of CINV and are included in these recommendations.

Choice of antiemetic agent. Many clinical institutions have pharmacy committees that provide recommendations or formularies for specific antiemetic regimens. These recommendations should be based on cost, efficacy and toxicity.

TABLE 4.3

Antiemetic agents and recommended doses to prevent CINV

Antiemetic	Oral dose	Intravenous dose
5-HT$_3$ RAs		
Ondansetron	24 mg	8 mg or 0.15 mg/kg (< 16 mg)
Granisetron	2 mg	1 mg or 0.01 mg/kg
Tropisetron	5 mg	5 mg
Dolasetron*	100 mg	100 mg or 0.18 mg/kg
Palonosetron	0.5 mg	0.25 mg
Dexamethasone	8–12 mg	8–12 mg
NK-1 RAs		
Aprepitant	125 mg on day 1	–
	80 mg days 2 and 3	
Fosaprepitant	–	150 mg on day 1
Rolapitant	180 mg	–
Netupitant/ palonosetron (NEPA)	300 mg/0.5 mg	–

*Not recommended in the USA because of QTc interval prolongation.

Choice of 5-HT$_3$ RA. There are no differences in efficacy between the first-generation 5-HT$_3$ RAs (dolasetron, granisetron, ondansetron and tropisetron), and all of the agents in this class have similar or minimal toxicity.

Two studies have compared the second-generation 5-HT$_3$ RA palonosetron with ondansetron and granisetron in the prevention of cisplatin-induced nausea and vomiting.[6,7] In the first trial, intravenous palonosetron, 0.25 mg and 0.75 mg, was compared with intravenous ondansetron, 32 mg.[6] In the second trial, palonosetron, 0.75 mg, was compared with granisetron, 40 µg/kg.[7] The two studies demonstrated that palonosetron induced better protection against delayed emesis, but did not discuss whether palonosetron was superior to other 5-HT$_3$ RAs when an NK-1 RA is used, as endorsed by current guidelines.

In addition, a meta-analysis of 16 randomized clinical trials compared palonosetron to the first-generation 5-HT$_3$ RAs. When administered without an NK-1 RA, palonosetron was statistically superior to the other 5-HT$_3$ RAs in its control of CINV in patients receiving both MEC and HEC. As discussed on page 34, this meta-analysis revealed that palonosetron is statistically superior in the acute, delayed and overall phases.[8]

Ondansetron, granisetron and (oral) dolasetron are available as generics; palonosetron is not available as a generic and has a higher acquisition cost. Tropisetron is distributed in various countries worldwide, but is not available in the USA.

International guidelines recommend the use of palonosetron as the preferred agent because of its higher efficacy compared with ondansetron or granisetron (see above). If the use of palonosetron results in better control of CINV with fewer visits to the clinic or the emergency department after chemotherapy and fewer admissions to the hospital for control of CINV, then its use may be cost-effective despite its initial higher acquisition cost.

Choice of NK-1 RA. Aprepitant, fosaprepitant, netupitant and rolapitant have all been shown to be safe and effective in phase III clinical trials, with few adverse events (see Chapter 3).

Aprepitant, fosaprepitant and netupitant are metabolized by the liver enzyme CYP3A4 and are moderate inhibitors of CYP3A4, potentially resulting in drug interactions, although few, if any, clinical adverse events attributable to CYP3A interactions have been reported. Rolapitant does not induce CYP3A4.

To date, no definitive clinical trials have directly compared the efficacy and safety of the various NK-1 RAs. One of the netupitant–palonosetron (NEPA) clinical trials involving patients receiving HEC included a comparative arm of oral aprepitant plus intravenous ondansetron. All patients in both arms received standard doses of dexamethasone. There appeared to be no significant differences in adverse events or in the prevention of CINV between NEPA and the aprepitant–ondansetron combination. A formal statistical comparison of the NEPA and aprepitant/ondansetron arms was not reported.[9] For the present, the choice among these agents may be based on cost and the availability of oral or intravenous forms.

Moderately emetogenic chemotherapy

Standard prophylactic control of acute and delayed CINV that may occur as a result of a non-AC MEC requires a combination of a 5-HT$_3$ RA (palonosetron is preferred) and dexamethasone administered before chemotherapy on day 1, followed by dexamethasone treatment on days 2–3 for the prevention of delayed nausea and vomiting (Figure 4.3).

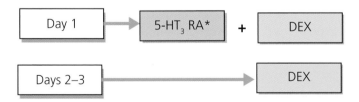

Figure 4.3 Guideline-directed treatment for acute and delayed CINV for patients receiving non-anthracycline–cyclophosphamide (AC)-based moderately emetogenic chemotherapy. *Palonosetron is the preferred agent for this indication.

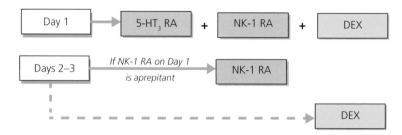

Figure 4.4 Guideline-directed treatment for acute and delayed CINV for patients receiving carboplatin-based moderately emetogenic chemotherapy. Some, but not all, clinicians advocate the use of dexamethasone on days 2–3.

Prophylactic control of carboplatin-based CINV requires a triple-drug combination of a NK-1 RA, a 5-HT$_3$ RA and dexamethasone before chemotherapy is administered on day 1. If aprepitant, 125 mg, is used on day 1, aprepitant, 80 mg, is recommended on days 2–3 for the prevention of delayed CINV. If another NK-1 RA is used on day 1, no additional NK-1 prophylaxis for delayed CINV prevention is recommended (Figure 4.4). At present there is no consensus as to whether to administer dexamethasone on days 2–3.

Prophylactic control of CINV induced by a multiple-day cisplatin regimen comprises a 5-HT$_3$ RA, dexamethasone and an NK-1 RA (aprepitant or fosaprepitant) for acute nausea and vomiting, and dexamethasone and an NK-1 RA (aprepitant or fosaprepitant) for delayed nausea and vomiting (Figure 4.5). However, it should be noted that there are only limited data on the use of aprepitant in this setting and, given the few studies to

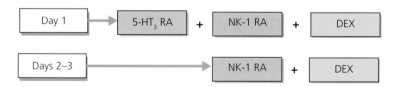

Figure 4.5 Guideline-directed treatment for acute and delayed CINV for patients receiving a multiple-day cisplatin chemotherapy regimen.

date in this patient population, the optimal doses of aprepitant and fosaprepitant still need to be determined. Some clinicians add 2 days of aprepitant to the regimen after completion of multiple-day chemotherapy to control the delayed nausea and vomiting that may occur after the final day of chemotherapy. There are no data for rolapitant or netupitant in patients receiving multiple-day cisplatin treatment, and the optimal doses of 5-HT$_3$ RA and dexamethasone have yet to be determined.

Furthermore, the 20-mg dose of dexamethasone that is often used on each day of chemotherapy has only been studied in patients receiving single-day higher doses of cisplatin-based chemotherapy ($\geq$ 50 mg/m^2). It is not known whether a lower dexamethasone dose administered on days 1–5 would be equivalent to a 20-mg dose.

Low or minimally emetogenic chemotherapy

Limited evidence from clinical studies support the choice of antiemetic therapy or of any treatment at all for patients receiving low or minimally emetogenic chemotherapy. Of the patients who receive low or minimally emetogenic chemotherapy, it is hard to categorize those at risk of developing nausea and vomiting.

Patients with no previous history of nausea and vomiting who undergo chemotherapy of low emetic potential as an intermittent schedule could be managed with a single antiemetic agent such as dexamethasone, a 5-HT$_3$ RA or a dopamine RA (Figure 4.6).

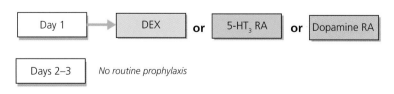

Figure 4.6 Guideline-directed treatment for acute and delayed CINV for patients receiving chemotherapy of low emetogenic potential. No routine prophylaxis is recommended for minimally emetogenic chemotherapy.

High-dose chemotherapy

Although the natural history of CINV in patients treated with high-dose chemotherapy and stem cell transplantation is, for the most part, unknown, most of these patients have experienced emesis with previous chemotherapy or irradiation.

The cause of CINV in this setting is multifactorial. Contributing causes include the use of prophylactic antibiotics, narcotic analgesics administered for the management of mucositis and total-body irradiation. Until recently, only phase II studies of antiemetic treatment with a 5-HT_3 RA alone or combined with dexamethasone had been carried out in these patients. A cross comparison of these trials was challenging given the various chemotherapy regimens employed, the duration of high-dose chemotherapy, and the different patient populations and tumor types involved. Furthermore, most of these trials were underpowered, included only a small number of patients, and had different clinical endpoints to those used in standard phase III antiemetic trials, making interpretation particularly challenging.

In recent years, phase III studies have been published that investigated the use of modern triple-antiemetic therapy consisting of a 5-HT_3 RA, dexamethasone and aprepitant. In a phase III study, 179 patients were randomized to receive ondansetron and dexamethasone with or without aprepitant on each day of the high-dose preparative regimen. A complete response (significant reduction in emesis without increasing toxicity or use of rescue medication) was demonstrated in 82% of those receiving aprepitant compared with 66% in those who did not.[10]

The efficacy of aprepitant has also been evaluated in a phase III study in patients with multiple myeloma undergoing a high-dose chemotherapy regimen of intravenous melphalan, 100 mg/m^2, on days 1–2, with autologous stem cell transplantation on day 4. The patients were randomized to receive either oral aprepitant, 125 mg, on day 1 followed by 80 mg on days 2–4, or oral granisetron, 2 mg, on days 1–4 with oral dexamethasone, 4 mg, on day 1 and 2 mg on days 2–3, or matching placebo with oral dexamethasone, 8 mg, on day 1 and 4 mg on days 2–3. A total of 362 patients were available for the efficacy analysis, with 181 in each treatment arm. The complete response rate was significantly greater in the aprepitant group than the control group (58% vs 41%).[11]

Key points – prevention and management of acute and delayed CINV

- The primary goal of CINV therapy is the prevention of nausea and vomiting.
- Patients should be individually evaluated for their specific risk factors as well as the level of anxiety present before the first course of treatment.
- Outcomes are improved by following international guidelines when selecting the antiemetic regimen to use in relation to emetogenicity of the type of chemotherapy involved.
- The triple-drug regimen of a NK-1 receptor antagonist (RA), 5-HT$_3$ RA and dexamethasone is recommended for patients receiving highly emetogenic chemotherapy.
- The two-drug combination of palonosetron and dexamethasone is recommended for patients receiving moderately emetogenic chemotherapy.
- A single 8-mg dose of dexamethasone before chemotherapy is recommended for patients receiving low emetogenic chemotherapy; no antiemetic should be administered routinely for patients receiving minimally emetogenic chemotherapy.
- The final choice of antiemetic agent will depend on efficacy, toxicity and cost. To determine overall cost-effectiveness of any given regimen, the acquisition cost of the antiemetic agent should be weighed against the probability and cost of post-chemotherapy visits to the clinic or emergency department and/or admissions to hospital.
- The incidence and severity of CINV in children is similar ito that in adults. The use of antiemetics in children should follow the same principles as those used to treat adults.

CINV in children

The incidence and severity of CINV in the pediatric age group is similar to that in adults.[12–14]

The use of antiemetics should follow the same principles as those used to treat adults. The literature on the use of specific agents for particular chemotherapy regimens in children is not as well developed as that in adults, mainly because the phase III clinical trials performed for the approval of 5-HT$_3$ and NK-1 RAs were performed in adults only.

The main antiemetics administered to children have been the 5-HT$_3$ RAs (ondansetron, granisetron, palonosetron) with or without the use of corticosteroids. The use of corticosteroids has depended on the risk:benefit ratio in specific age groups and the particular chemotherapy regimen being used.[12]

Recently, aprepitant has been recommended for use in various age groups and various clinical applications.[14,15] To date, there have been no studies in children with netupitant or rolapitant.

Key references

1. MASCC/ESMO Antiemetic Guidelines. www.mascc.org/antiemetic-guidelines, last accessed 15 March 2016.

Gralla RJ, Roila F, Tonato M, Herrstedt J. MASCC/ESMO Antiemetic Guideline 2013. www.mascc.org/assets/Guidelines-Tools/mascc_antiemetic_english_2014.pdf.

Roila F, Herrstedt J, Aapro M et al.; ESMO/MASCC Guidelines Working Group. Guideline update for MASCC and ESMO in the prevention of chemotherapy and radiotherapy-induced nausea and vomiting: results of the Perugia consensus conference. Ann Oncol 2010;21(Suppl5):232–43.

2. Hesketh PJ, Bohike K, Lyman GH et al. Antiemetics: American Society of Clinical Oncology focused guideline update. J Clin Oncol 2016;34:381–6.

3. Basch E, Prestrud AA, Hesketh PJ et al. Antiemetics: American Society of Clinical Oncology clinical practice guideline update. J Clin Oncol 2011;29:4189–98.

4. NCCN. Guidelines for Supportive Care: Antiemesis. National Comprehensive Cancer Network www.nccn.org/professionals/physician_gls/f_guidelines.asp#supportive.

5. Gilmore JW, Peacock NW, Gu A, et al. Antiemetic guideline consistency and incidence of chemotherapy-induced nausea and vomiting in US community oncology practice: INSPIRE study. *J Oncol Pract* 2014;10:68–74.

6. Aapro MS, Grunberg SM, Manikhas GM et al. A phase III, double-blind, randomized trial of palonosetron compared with ondansetron in preventing chemotherapy-induced nausea and vomiting following highly emetogenic chemotherapy. *Ann Oncol* 2006;17:1441–9.

7. Saito M, Aogi K, Sekine I et al. Palonosetron plus dexamethasone versus granisetron plus dexamethasone for prevention of nausea and vomiting during chemotherapy: a double-blind, double-dummy, randomised, comparative phase III trial. *Lancet Oncol* 2009;10:115–24.

8. Popovic M, Warr DG, Deangelis C et al. Efficacy and safety of palonosetron for the prophylaxis of chemotherapy-induced nausea and vomiting (CINV): a systematic review and meta-analysis of randomized controlled trials. *Support Care Cancer* 2014;22:1685–97.

9. Hesketh PJ, Rossi G, Rizzi G et al. Efficacy and safety of NEPA, an oral combination of netupitant and palonosetron, for prevention of chemotherapy-induced nausea and vomiting following highly emetogenic chemotherapy: a randomized dose-ranging pivotal study. *Ann Oncol* 2014;25:1340–6.

10. Stiff PJ, Fox-Geiman MP, Kiley K et al. Prevention of nausea and vomiting associated with stem cell transplant: results of a prospective, randomized trial of aprepitant used with highly emetogenic preparative regimens. *Biol Blood Marrow Transplant* 2013;19:49–55e.

11. Schmitt T, Goldschmidt H, Neben K et al. Aprepitant, granisetron, and dexamethasone for prevention of chemotherapy-induced nausea and vomiting after high-dose melphalan in autologous transplantation for multiple myeloma: results of a randomized, placebo-controlled phase III trial. *J Clin Oncol* 2014;32:3413–20.

12. Patel P, Robinson PD, Orsey A et al. Chemotherapy-induced nausea and vomiting prophylaxis: practice within the Children's Oncology Group. *Pediatr Blood Cancer* 2016;Jan 27 [Epub ahead of print].

13. Phillips RS, Friend AJ, Gibson F et al. Antiemetic medication for prevention and treatment of chemotherapy-induced nausea and vomiting in childhood. *Cochrane Database Syst Rev* 2016;2:CD007786. [Epub ahead of print].

14. Dupuis LL, Boodhan S, Holdsworth M et al. Guideline for the prevention of acute nausea and vomiting due to antineoplastic medication in pediatric cancer patients. *Pediatr Blood Cancer* 2013;60:1073–82.

15. Kang HJ, Loftus S, Taylor A et al. Aprepitant for the prevention of chemotherapy-induced nausea and vomiting in children: a randomized, double-blind, phase 3 trial. *Lancet Oncol* 2015;16:385–94.

Further reading

Aapro M, Molassiotis A, Dicato M et al. The effect of guideline-consistent antiemetic therapy on chemotherapy-induced nausea and vomiting (CINV): the Pan European Emesis Registry (PEER). *Ann Oncol* 2012;23:1986–92.

Jordan K, Gralla R, Jahn F, Molassiotis A. International antiemetic guidelines on chemotherapy induced nausea and vomiting (CINV): content and implementation in daily routine practice. *Eur J Pharmacol* 2014;722:197–202.

Schmitt T, Goldschmidt H, Neben K, et al. Aprepitant, granisetron, and dexamethasone for prevention of chemotherapy-induced nausea and vomiting after high-dose melphalan in autologous transplantation for multiple myeloma: results of a randomized, placebo-controlled phase III trial. *J Clin Oncol* 2014;21:3413–20.

Breakthrough CINV

Even with improved control of acute and delayed CINV and adequate antiemetic prophylaxis, breakthrough CINV within 5 days of chemotherapy administration (see page 17) remains a significant clinical problem.

Management principles. Breakthrough CINV usually requires immediate treatment or 'rescue' with additional antiemetics. Clinicians should provide patients with a prescription for rescue antiemetic treatment before the patient leaves the clinic or hospital, so that in the event of breakthrough CINV occurring, treatment can be started immediately. As patients may or may not derive some benefit from the original antiemetic regimen, this may or may not be continued.

It is very unlikely that breakthrough nausea and vomiting will respond to an agent in the same drug class, and therefore with the same mechanism of action, as that already used unsuccessfully for prophylaxis. Agents that are found to effectively treat a patient's breakthrough CINV should be given routinely for at least 3 days rather than on an as-needed basis.[1-4]

Treatment options. Antiemetic treatment options recommended by the Multinational Association for Supportive Care in Cancer (MASCC) and the American Society of Clinical Oncology (ASCO) are illustrated in Table 5.1.[1-4]

The US National Comprehensive Cancer Network (NCCN) guidelines suggest treating breakthrough CINV with an agent from a drug class that was not used in the prophylactic regimen and recommend continuing the breakthrough medication if nausea and vomiting is controlled with that specific agent.[4]

TABLE 5.1

Antiemetic options for treatment of breakthrough CINV

- Olanzapine, 10 mg, PO, daily
- Dexamethasone, 4 mg, PO, twice a day
- Prochlorperazine, 10 mg, PO, every 4–8 hours
- Haloperidol, 0.5 mg, PO, twice a day
- Benzodiazepines:
  - Lorazepam, 0.5–1.0 mg, PO, daily
  - Alprazolam, 0.25 mg, PO, twice a day
  - Diazepam, 5 mg, PO, daily
- Metoclopramide, 10 mg, PO, three times a day
- A 5-HT$_3$ receptor antagonist, provided that a 5-HT$_3$ receptor antagonist was not used in the prophylactic regimen

The agents used prophylactically to prevent CINV have not demonstrated significant efficacy in the treatment of established CINV.[5] Olanzapine and metoclopramide have been the only agents studied for the treatment of breakthrough CINV in phase III clinical trials.[6,7]

In a phase III clinical trial involving 80 patients on highly emetogenic chemotherapy (HEC), a 3-day regimen of oral olanzapine, 10 mg/day, was shown to be superior to 3 days of oral metoclopramide, 10 mg 3 times daily. During 72 hours of observation, significantly more patients receiving olanzapine had no recurrent emesis (70% vs 31%) and no nausea (68% vs 23%).[7] On this basis, the NCCN guidelines state that patients who develop nausea or vomiting after chemotherapy (days 1 to 5) despite adequate prophylaxis should be considered for treatment with a 3-day regimen of oral olanzapine, 10 mg/day.

Despite the lack of phase III clinical trials, current guidelines also suggest the use of a phenothiazine, metoclopramide, dexamethasone, dopamine antagonists (e.g. prochlorperazine, haloperidol), benzodiazepines, an anticholinergic, or olanzapine. A 5-HT$_3$ receptor antagonist (RA) may also be effective unless a patient presents with breakthrough nausea and vomiting that developed after the use of a 5-HT$_3$ RA as prophylaxis for chemotherapy or radiotherapy-induced emesis (see Table 5.1).

It is important to note that although the neurokinin-1 (NK-1) receptor antagonists (aprepitant, fosaprepitant, netupitant, rolapitant) have been approved as additive agents to a 5-HT$_3$ receptor antagonist and dexamethasone for the prevention of CINV, they have not been studied and should not be used to treat breakthrough nausea and vomiting.[5]

Refractory CINV

A change in the prophylactic antiemetic regimen should be considered for those patients who develop CINV during subsequent cycles of chemotherapy when antiemetic prophylaxis has not been successful in controlling CINV in earlier cycles.

Treatment options. Few studies have examined CINV in this setting. If anxiety is considered to be a major patient factor in CINV, a benzodiazepine such as lorazepam or alprazolam can be added to the prophylactic regimen.

If the patient is receiving HEC, olanzapine (days 1 to 4) can be substituted for the NK-1 RA in the prophylactic antiemetic regimen.[8–10] The best available evidence suggests the use of oral olanzapine, 10 mg for 3 days.[7] Mild to moderate sedation in elderly patients may be a potential problem associated with olanzapine.

If the patient is receiving moderately emetogenic chemotherapy (MEC), aprepitant or fosaprepitant can be added to the palonosetron and dexamethasone antiemetic regimen.[11] NCCN guidelines recommend the use of olanzapine, palonosetron and dexamethasone as an alternative first-line prophylactic antiemetic regimen for patients receiving HEC. This regimen may be useful in patients who experience refractory CINV and need a revision in their prophylactic antiemetic regimen.[4,8]

Non-pharmacological interventions such as acupuncture could also be considered, although there is no clear evidence with regards to efficacy.

Anticipatory CINV

If CINV is effectively controlled during the first cycle of chemotherapy, the patient is likely to have effective control during subsequent cycles of the same chemotherapy. If the patient has a poor experience with CINV in the first cycle, it may be more difficult to control CINV in subsequent cycles, and refractory and/or anticipatory CINV may develop.

The earlier anticipatory CINV is identified, the more likely treatment will be effective.

Management principles. To prevent the occurrence of anticipatory CINV (see pages 17–18), patients should be counseled about their 'expectations' of CINV before the initial course of treatment. Patients should be informed that very effective prophylactic antiemetic regimens will be used and that 70–75% of patients have a complete response (i.e. no emesis and no use of rescue medications). For optimum control of CINV during the first course of chemotherapy, each patient should receive the most effective prophylactic antiemetic regimen based on the specific type of chemotherapy (see Tables 4.1 and 4.2, pages 54–7) and their individual risk factors (see Table 2.2, page 18) before the first course of chemotherapy.

Treatment options. The use of anti-anxiety medications such as lorazepam or another benzodiazepine may be considered for excess anxiety prior to the first course of chemotherapy in order to obtain an optimum outcome and prevent anticipatory CINV. If anticipatory CINV occurs despite the use of guideline-directed prophylactic antiemetics, additional antiemetic drugs do not seem to be effective. Behavioral therapy should be considered instead. A number of behavioral interventions have been investigated (Table 5.2).[12–16]

Progressive muscle relaxation with guided imagery, hypnosis, and systematic desensitization have been studied the most and are potential treatment options. Early screening and referral to a psychologist or other mental health professional with specific experience of working with patients with cancer is essential when anticipatory CINV is identified.

TABLE 5.2

Behavioral interventions for anticipatory CINV

- Progressive muscle relaxation with guided imagery
- Hypnosis
- Systematic desensitization
- Electromyography and thermal biofeedback
- Distraction via the use of video games

Key points – treatment of breakthrough, refractory and anticipatory CINV

- Breakthrough CINV within 5 days of chemotherapy administration remains a significant clinical problem despite the development of effective agents for the prevention of CINV. Olanzapine has been shown in a phase III clinical trial to be an effective treatment.
- A change in the prophylactic antiemetic regimen should be considered for those patients who develop refractory CINV.
- If the patient has a poor experience with CINV in the first cycle, anticipatory CINV may develop requiring behavioral therapy.
- Optimum control of CINV during the first course of chemotherapy may prevent breakthrough, refractory and anticipatory CINV. Each patient should receive the most effective prophylactic antiemetic regimen based on the specific type of chemotherapy and their individual risk factors before the first course of chemotherapy.

Key references

1. Roila F, Herrstedt J, Aapro M et al. Guideline update for MASCC and ESMO in the prevention of chemotherapy- and radiotherapy-induced nausea and vomiting: results of the Perugia consensus conference. *Ann Oncol* 2010;21:232–43.

2. Basch E, Prestrud AA, Hesketh PJ et al. Antiemetic American Society Clinical Oncology clinical practice guideline update. *J Clin Oncol* 2011;29:4189–98.

3. Hesketh PJ, Bohike K, Lyman GH et al. Antiemetics: American Society of Clinical Oncology focused guideline update. *J Clin Oncol* 2015; DOI: JCO 2015.64.3635s.

4. NCCN Clinical Practice Guidelines in Oncology version 2.2014; Antiemesis. National Comprehensive Cancer Network (NCCN) [online]. www.nccn.org/professionals/physician_gls/PDF/antiemesis.pdf, last accessed 08 November 2015.

5. Kris MC. Why do we need another antiemetic? Just ask. *J Clin Oncol* 2003;21:4077–80.

6. www.cancer.gov/cancertopics/pdq/supportivecare/nausea/healthprofessional

7. Navari RM, Nagy CK, Gray SE. The use of olanzapine versus metoclopramide for the treatment of breakthrough chemotherapy-induced nausea and vomiting in patients receiving highly emetogenic chemotherapy. *Support Care Cancer* 2013;21:1655–63.

8. Navari RM, Gray SE, Kerr AC. Olanzapine versus aprepitant for the prevention of chemotherapy-induced nausea and vomiting: A randomized phase III trial. *J Support Oncol* 2011;9:188–95.

9. Vig S, Seibert L, Green MR. Olanzapine is effective for refractory chemotherapy-induced nausea and vomiting irrespective of chemotherapy emetogenicity. *J Cancer Res Clin Oncol* 2014;140:77–82.

10. Bradford MV, Glode A. Olanzapine: an antiemetic option for chemotherapy-induced nausea and vomiting. *J Adv Pract Oncol* 2014;5:24–9.

11. Rapoport BL, Jordon K, Boice JA et al. Aprepitant for the prevention of chemotherapy-induced nausea and vomiting associated with a broad range of moderately emetogenic chemotherapies and tumor types: a randomized, double-blind study. *Support Care Cancer* 2010;18:423–31.

12. Lyles JN, Burish TG, Krozely MG et al. Efficacy of relaxation training and guided imagery in reducing the aversiveness of cancer chemotherapy. *J Consult Clin Psychol* 1982;50:509–24.

13. Redd WH, Andresen GV, Minagawa RY. Hypnotic control of anticipatory emesis in patients receiving cancer chemotherapy. *J Consult Clin Psychol* 1982; 50:14–19.

14. Morrow GR, Morrell C. Behavioral treatment for the anticipatory nausea and vomiting induced by cancer chemotherapy. *N Engl J Med* 1982;307:1476–80.

15. Burish TG, Shartner CD, Lyles JN. Effectiveness of multiple muscle-site EMG biofeedback and relaxation training in reducing the aversiveness of cancer chemotherapy. *Biofeedback Self Regul* 1981;6: 523–35.

16. Kolko DJ, Rickard-Figueroa JL. Effects of video games on the adverse corollaries of chemotherapy in pediatric oncology patients: a single-case analysis. *J Consult Clin Psychol* 1985;53:223–8.

Further reading

Navari RM. Treatment of breakthrough and refractory chemotherapy-induced nausea and vomiting. *Biomed Res Int* 2015;2015:595894.

Pharmacological management

Conventional antiemetics are more successful at preventing emesis than nausea. Current data from multiple large studies suggest that neither first- nor second-generation 5-hydroxytryptamine-3 (5-HT$_3$) receptor antagonists (RAs) are effective in the control of nausea in patients receiving either moderately or highly emetogenic chemotherapy (MEC or HEC, respectively), despite marked improvement in the control of emesis.[2–5] Multiple large phase III trials have also shown that although the neurokinin (NK)-1 RA aprepitant is effective for the control of emesis, it is not effective in controling nausea in patients receiving MEC or HEC.[6] Similarly, phase III clinical trial data indicate that the new neurokinin (NK)-1 RAs netupitant and rolapitant are not effective antinausea agents,[7,8] although rolapitant may have some effect in patients receiving cisplatin HEC.[8]

These studies suggest that the serotonin (5-HT$_3$) and substance P (NK-1) receptors may not be important in the mediation of nausea, despite their important role in chemotherapy-induced emesis (see page 11).[2–5] New studies using novel agents and using nausea as the primary endpoint need to be performed.

Olanzapine appears to have high potential for the control of both emesis and nausea in patients receiving MEC or HEC (Table 6.1). Phase III studies suggest that olanzapine may be an important agent in the control of chemotherapy-induced nausea.[9–12] Olanzapine is known to affect a wide variety of receptors including dopamine D$_2$, 5-HT$_{2C}$, histaminic and muscarinic receptors. At present, there is still a substantial lack of understanding of the pathogenesis of chemotherapy-induced nausea, and any or all of these receptors may be important mediators.

TABLE 6.1

Pharmacological management of chemotherapy-induced nausea

	Treatment options
Acute CINV (0–24 hours)	Day 1:
	5-HT$_3$ RA (ondansetron, granisetron or palonosetron)* + NK-1 RA (aprepitant, fosaprepitant, netupitant or rolapitant)* + dexamethasone*
	or
	Olanzapine, 10 mg, PO, + 5-HT$_3$ RA (ondansetron, granisetron or palonosetron)* + dexamethasone*
	or
	Olanzapine, 10 mg, PO + 5-HT$_3$ RA (ondansetron, granisetron, or palonosetron)* + NK-1 RA (aprepitant, fosaprepitant, netupitant or rolapitant)* + dexamethasone*
Delayed CINV (24–120 hours)	Days 2–4:
	Olanzapine, 10 mg, PO daily
	or
	Olanzapine, 10 mg, PO daily + dexamethasone, daily*
Established nausea	Olanzapine, 10 mg, PO daily for 3 days

*See Table 4.3 for doses of various agents. 5-HT$_3$, 5-hydroxytrypatmine 3; CINV, chemotherapy-induced nausea and vomiting; NK-1, neurokinin-1; PO, per os (by mouth/oral); RA, receptor antagonist.

The addition of olanzapine to the 5-HT$_3$ RA azasetron and dexamethasone has been shown to improve nausea and emesis compared with azasetron and dexamethasone alone in patients receiving MEC and HEC.[9] Olanzapine, palonosetron and dexamethasone has been shown to improve the control of nausea compared with aprepitant, palonosetron and dexamethasone in patients receiving HEC.[10] Breakthrough nausea and emesis was controlled with olanzapine in patients receiving HEC and guideline-directed prophylactic antiemetics.[11] The addition of olanzapine to aprepitant, a 5-HT$_3$ RA and dexamethasone significantly improved nausea and emesis compared with aprepitant, a 5-HT$_3$ RA and dexamethasone alone in patients receiving HEC.[12] Olanzapine is available as a generic.

Other agents. Preliminary small studies with gabapentin have demonstrated some effectiveness in the control of chemotherapy-induced emesis, but the control of nausea has yet to be determined.[2] More studies with the use of cannabinoids need to be performed before it is known whether this class of agent is clinically efficacious in the control of CINV.[2] The studies performed to date do not support the use of ginger as an effective agent in the prevention of CINV.[2]

Non-pharmacological management

Few randomized clinical trials have demonstrated efficacy of non-pharmacological measures to prevent or treat chemotherapy-induced nausea. Table 6.2 summarizes measures suggested by case reports.

TABLE 6.2

Non-pharmacological management of chemotherapy-induced nausea

- Avoid strong odors in food or in your environment
- Eat small amounts of non-spicy, cold food frequently throughout the day
- Avoid caffeine and smoking
- Acupuncture

Key points – prevention and treatment of chemotherapy-induced nausea

- Current data from multiple large studies suggest that neither the 5-HT$_3$ receptor antagonists (RAs) nor the NK-1 RAs are effective in the prevention of nausea in patients receiving either moderately or highly emetogenic chemotherapy, despite marked improvement in the control of emesis.
- Phase III clinical studies suggest that olanzapine may be an important agent in the prevention of chemotherapy-induced nausea and in the treatment of breakthrough CINV.
- Non-pharmacological measures for the control of chemotherapy-induced nausea include avoidance of strong odors, eating small amounts of spicy food, avoiding smoking and caffeine, and acupuncture.

Key references

1. Stern RM, Koch KL, Andrews PLR. *Nausea: Mechanisms and Management.* New York: Oxford University Press, 2011.

2. Navari RM. Management of chemotherapy-induced nausea and vomiting: focus on new agents and new uses for older agents. *Drugs* 2013;73:249–62.

3. Navari RM. Treatment of chemotherapy-induced nausea. *Community Oncol* 2012;9:20–6.

4. Ng TL, Hutton B, Clemons M. Chemotherapy-induced nausea and vomiting: time for more emphasis on nausea? *Oncologist* 2015;20:576–83.

5. Navari RM. Olanzapine for the prevention and treatment of chronic nausea and chemotherapy-induced nausea and vomiting. *European J Pharm* 2014;722:180–6.

6. Aapro M, Carides A, Rapoport BL et al. Aprepitant and fosaprepitant: a 10-year review of efficacy and safety. *Oncologist* 2015;20:450–8.

7. Navari RM. Profile of netupitant/palonosetron fixed dose combination (NEPA) and its potential in the treatment of chemotherapy-induced nausea and vomiting (CINV). *Drug Des Devel Ther* 2015;9:155–61.

8. Navari RM. Rolapitant for the treatment of chemotherapy induced nausea and vomiting. *Expert Rev Anticancer Ther* 2015;15:1127–33.

9. Tan L, Liu J, Liu X et al. Clinical research of olanzapine for the prevention of chemotherapy-induced nausea and vomiting. *J Exp Clin Cancer Res* 2009;25:1–7.

10. Navari RM, Gray SE, Kerr AC. Olanzapine versus aprepitant for the prevention of chemotherapy induced nausea and vomiting (CINV): A randomized phase III trial. *J Supp Oncol* 2011;9:188–95.

11. Navari RM. Treatment of breakthrough and refractory chemotherapy-induced nausea and vomiting. *Biomed Res Int* 2015;2015:595894.

12. Navari RM, Qin R, Ruddy KJ et al. Olanzapine for the prevention of chemotherapy-induced nausea and vomiting in patients receiving highly emetogenic chemotherapy: Alliance A221301, a randomized, double-blind, placebo-controlled trial. ASCO Palliative Care Symposium, 2015; abstract 176, Boston.

Further reading

Roscoe JA, Heckler CE, Morrow GR et al. Prevention of delayed nausea: a University of Rochester Cancer Center Community Clinical Oncology Program study of patients receiving chemotherapy. *J Clin Oncol* 2012;30:3389–95.

7 Barriers and opportunities in CINV management

Barriers to CINV prevention and control

Despite clear international guidelines on the optimal use of antiemetic regimens for the prevention and control of chemotherapy-induced nausea and vomiting (CINV), these symptoms are still estimated to affect 35–50% of patients who undergo chemotherapy even with the use of effective antiemetic agents. Several issues continue to limit the effectiveness of CINV prevention and management:

- underestimation of the incidence of CINV by healthcare professionals and/or the effect it has on patients' quality of life
- concerns about the adverse effects and/or costs of antiemetic treatments
- lack of monitoring of patients in the 5 days immediately following chemotherapy
- under-reporting of the incidence of CINV by patients
- poor adherence to prescribed antiemetic medications.

Underestimating incidence and effect. A recent multinational European survey, aimed at verifying the incidence of CINV and the corresponding antiemetic treatment patterns, showed there is a perceptual gap between patients and physicians/oncology nurses, particularly in terms of the occurrence of nausea and the impact CINV has on patients' quality of life.[1] In total, 947 individuals (375 physicians, 186 oncology nurses and 386 patients) participated in the survey. Sixty percent of patients reported experiencing nausea only, 14% reported nausea and vomiting, and 4% reported vomiting only. Nausea without vomiting has only recently been thought of as a condition in its own right, and as such the incidence of nausea may often be underestimated. Although, in this survey, the physicians and oncology nurses overestimated the incidence of CINV, they underestimated its effect on patients' quality of life.

Prescribing concerns. In total, 76% of the physicians in the European survey described above prescribed guideline-directed CINV prophylaxis for patients receiving highly emetogenic chemotherapy (HEC). This decreased to 15% for moderately emetogenic chemotherapy (MEC), while 86% prescribed no or minimal antiemetic medication for patients receiving low emetogenic chemotherapy. Adverse effects and costs were cited as key factors in their reluctance to prescribe prophylactic CINV medication.

Lack of follow-up. No patient monitoring in the 5-day period following chemotherapy was reported by 27% of physicians and 33% of oncology nurses, and was confirmed by half of the patients.

Under-reporting by patients. The main reason for not reporting CINV in the European survey was a general perception by 51% of patients that nausea and vomiting is an inevitable consequence of chemotherapy that had to be tolerated. In another study, 37% of patients said they wanted 'to be strong by not complaining' about their symptoms.[2]

Poor adherence. Only 38% of patients in the European survey reported full adherence to the guidelines given to them by their physicians/oncology nurses when self-administering antiemetic medication. One reason cited for this poor adherence was 'not accepting the need to take medication until actually feeling sick'. Other factors included reluctance to add to the pill burden and fear that swallowing itself would induce nausea/vomiting.

Opportunties for improving CINV prevention and control

There are a number of institutional or clinic operational procedures that may address the issues above, and improve the quality of care of patients receiving chemotherapy.

Better prescribing. Incorporating antiemetic guidelines in electronic medical record prescribing orders may help to ensure prescription of optimal antiemetic regimens. Studies have shown that oncology nurses and nurse practitioners can have a key role in influencing the selection of the antiemetic regimen, and it is important that they are aware of the latest antiemetic guidelines and the factors that put patients at risk for CINV.[3] In a multidisciplinary team, communication between oncology nurses, palliative care nurses, pharmacists and clinicians about the antiemetic regimen and the patient's progress is essential.

Patient education. Clinicians should reassure patients that the incidence or severity of CINV is not an indicator of the effectiveness of their chemotherapy and that nausea and vomiting should not be considered a normal part of treatment. Furthermore, it is important to discuss the likelihood and management of adverse effects of antiemetic treatment and emphasize the importance of continuing the medications at home and completing the full course of treatment. Minimizing the pill burden and eliminating the requirement to swallow medication can also improve patient adherence to treatment.

Improved follow-up. It is important to assess symptoms throughout therapy, as patient response to antiemetic treatment may change over time and may require adjustment of the antiemetic regimen. Telephone follow-up by oncology nurses with patients 24–48 hours after chemotherapy will provide important patient information as well as suggested treatment for unreported breakthrough CINV.

Future research. At present, olanzapine appears to be the only current effective agent for the control of nausea (see Chapter 6). Despite the control of emesis with the 5-HT$_3$ RAs, dexamethasone and the NK-1 RAs, nausea remains an important and prevalent clinical issue. Given the high incidence of nausea only experienced by patients, a better understanding of the pathophysiology of nausea and new approaches to its treatment are required.

Key points – barriers and opportunities in CINV management

- Issues that may reduce the effectiveness of CINV control by healthcare professionals include underestimation of the incidence of CINV, concerns about the adverse effects and cost of antiemetic agents, and insufficient following up after chemotherapy.
- Patient factors that may reduce the effectiveness of CINV control include under-reporting of symptoms and poor adherence to medications.
- Incorporating antiemetic guidelines in electronic medical record prescribing orders may help to ensure prescription of optimal antiemetic regimens by healthcare professionals.
- Clinicians must emphasize the importance of continuing medications at home and completing the full course of treatment.
- Telephone follow-up by oncology nurses with patients 24–48 hours after chemotherapy will provide important patient information.

Key references

1. Vidall C, Fernandez-Ortega P, Cortinovis D et al. Impact and management of chemotherapy/radiotherapy-induced nausea and vomiting and the perceptual gap between oncologists/oncology nurses and patients: a cross-sectional multinational survey. *Support Care Cancer* 2015;23:3297–305.

2. Salsman JM, Grunberg SM, Beaumont JL et al. Communicating about chemotherapy-induced nausea and vomiting: a comparison of patient and provider perspectives. *J Natl Compr Canc Netw* 2012;10:149–57.

3. Rogers MP, Blackburn L. Use of neurokinin-1 receptor antagonists in patients receiving moderately or highly emetogenic chemotherapy. *Clin J Oncol Nurs* 2010;14:500–4.

Further reading

Dranitsaris G, Leung P, Warr D. Implementing evidence based antiemetic guidelines in the oncology setting: results of a 4-month prospective intervention study. *Support Care Cancer* 2001;9: 611–18.

Mertens WC, Higby DJ, Brown D et al. Improving the care of patients with regard to chemotherapy-induced nausea and emesis: the effect of feedback to clinicians on adherence to antiemetic prescribing guidelines. *J Clin Oncol* 2003;21:1373–8.

Molassiotis A, Saunders MP, Valle J et al. A prospective observational study of chemotherapy-related nausea and vomiting in routine practice in a UK cancer centre. *Support Care Cancer* 2008;16: 201–8.

Roila F. Transferring scientific evidence to oncological practice: a trial on the impact of three different implementation strategies on antiemetic prescriptions. *Support Care Cancer* 2004;12:446–53.

Yu S, Burke TA, Chan A et al. Antiemetic therapy in Asia Pacific countries for patients receiving moderately and highly emetogenic chemotherapy – a descriptive analysis of practice patterns, antiemetic quality of care, and use of antiemetic guidelines. *Support Care Cancer* 2015;23:273–82.

Useful resources

American Society of Oncology
Tel (CME): +1 571 483 1403
cme@asco.org
Patient info: +1 571 483 1780
contactus@cancer.net
Conquer Cancer Foundation
Tel: +1 571 483 1700
info@conquercancerfoundation.org
www.asco.org

European Society for Medical Oncology
Tel: +41 (0)91 973 19 00
esmo@esmo.org
www.esmo.org

Multinational Association of Supportive Care in Cancer
Tel: +45 4820 7022
aschultz@mascc.org
www.mascc.org

National Cancer Institute (USA)
Helpline: 1 800 422 6237
www.cancer.gov

National Comprehensive Cancer Network (USA)
Tel: +1 215 690 0300
www.nccn.org

Guidelines
Basch E, Prestrud AA, Hesketh PJ et al. Antiemetics: American Society of Clinical Oncology clinical practice guideline update. *J Clin Oncol* 2011;29:4189–98.

Hesketh PJ, Bohike K, Lyman GH et al. Antiemetics: American Society of Clinical Oncology focused guideline update. *J Clin Oncol* 2016;34:381–6.

Multinational Association of Supportive Care in Cancer/ESMO Antiemetic Guideline 2013. www.mascc.org/antiemetic-guidelines

NCCN Clinical Practice Guidelines in Oncology version 2.2014; Antiemesis. National Comprehensive Cancer Network www.nccn.org/ professionals/physician_gls/PDF/antiemesis.pdf

Roila F, Herrstedt J, Aapro M et al. Guideline update for MASCC and ESMO in the prevention of chemotherapy and radiotherapy-induced nausea and vomiting: results of the Perugia consensus conference. *Ann Oncol* 2010;21(Suppl5):232–43.

Index